SAFE BLOOD

SAFE BLOOD

Purifying the Nation's Blood Supply in the Age of AIDS

Joseph Feldschuh, M.D.
with
Doron Weber

THE FREE PRESS
A Division of Macmillan, Inc.
NEW YORK

Collier Macmillan Canada
TORONTO

Maxwell Macmillan International
NEW YORK   OXFORD   SINGAPORE   SYDNEY

The Free Press
A Division of Macmillan, Inc.
866 Third Avenue, New York, N.Y. 10022

Collier Macmillan Canada, Inc.
1200 Eglinton Avenue East
Suite 200
Don Mills, Ontario M3C 3N1

Printed in the United States of America

printing number
1 2 3 4 5 6 7 8 9 10

Library of Congress Cataloging-in-Publication Data
Feldschuh, Joseph.
    Safe blood : purifying the nation's blood supply in the age of
AIDS / Joseph Feldschuh with Doron Weber.
        p.   cm.
    ISBN 0-68-486386-3
    1. Blood—transfusion—Safety measures.   2. Blood banks—Quality
control.   3. Health risk factors.   I. Weber, Doron.   II. Title.
        [DNLM]:   1. Blood Banks.   2. Blood Transfusions.   3. Quality
Control.   4. Risk Factors.   WB 356 F312s]
    RM171.F43   1990
362.1'784'0973—dc20
DNLM/DLC
for Library of Congress   89–23758
                                                CIP

Contents

Preface

The origins of this book go back to a quiet day in October 1959, when a young medical student sitting in anatomy class at New York University Medical School was suddenly called out of the classroom. There is a special anxiety and dread that grips people when their routine is suddenly disrupted; they *know* something bad is about to happen.

The student was informed that his father had collapsed in Grand Central Station and had been rushed to the emergency room of Bellevue Hospital. The father had hemorrhaged from a bleeding ulcer and had lost considerable amounts of blood. His condition had been stabilized with blood substitutes, but he was clearly going to require transfusions in order to survive.

The son quickly offered to donate his own blood and recruited three of his classmates with similar blood types to donate theirs. In 1959, minimal testing was performed on blood, and over a 48-hour period the father was successfully transfused with four pints of blood.

Such was my personal initiation into the world of blood transfusion and my introduction to the blood banking system. My knowledge of transfusion was extremely limited at the time, although I was vaguely aware that there were some possible dangers. Over the next 29 years, my father was to receive a total of 20 pints of blood (11 donated by me) on six separate occasions for a number of medical and surgical conditions, and I was to become intimately acquainted with all the benefits, as well as the dangers, of transfusion. Had the blood transfusion system not been in existence, my father's life would have ended in 1959. However, had there been a better system, my father might still be alive today.

Six years after his initial episode, my father hemorrhaged again

viii   Preface

and received further transfusions. After one of them he developed a severe, shaking reaction. It seems that as a result of his previous transfusions, my father had developed antibodies to one of the numerous human blood subtypes. These antibodies now brought on an allergic reaction to the new, incompatible blood he had received, blood that was being attacked and destroyed inside his body.

My father was in a precarious state. He required a transfusion, but it was very difficult to give him additional blood because a similar reaction might occur. I had already given him a unit of my own blood and pleaded with the doctors to take a second pint from me. The best chance of a close match is between blood relatives; my father had previously been exposed to my blood, so I knew we were compatible.

However, the hospital guidelines stipulated that a donor could give no more than one pint of blood in an eight-week period.* Despite my pleading, the offer to donate additional blood was refused, and a mad scramble ensued to find a safe unit of blood before my father's blood pressure sank too low. Fortunately such a unit was located, and my father's life was saved.

On that day in 1964, I learned that there are hundreds of blood subtypes in addition to the basic ABO groups and that the chances of getting an exact, matching blood transfusion from a total stranger are less than 1 in 100,000. I will never forget the helpless feeling that overcame me at the thought that my father might die because he could not get safe, matching blood.

I now embarked on a study of the blood banking situation, and what I found shocked and dismayed me. My first realization, of course, was that blood typing is not as simple as I had always assumed. I learned that it is very common for people to have minor reactions from transfused blood because of incompatibilities between donor and recipient. Occasionally, these incompatibilities could result in a severe transfusion reaction, as in my father's case. In even more drastic circumstances, where, for example, type A blood is mistakenly given to a type B person, death is very likely.

I also discovered that hepatitis infections are a relatively common consequence of blood transfusion, a risk of which the public and most physicians seemed unaware. Yet most studies at the time suggested that at least one in ten individuals who received a transfusion developed hepatitis, an alarming rate considering that several million Americans each year needed a blood transfusion.

*This eight-week guideline was subsequently adopted by the Food and Drug Administration (FDA) and has been official policy for many years.

I was grateful to a system that had saved my father's life. But mindful of his severe reaction and the other disturbing facts I had unearthed, I wondered if there were not a better way to supply blood to those who needed it; at that time, I made a promise to myself that if I were ever in a position to reform and improve the system, I would do it.

In 1966, after completing two successive fellowships in endocrinology and cardiology, respectively, I accepted a half-time teaching position at New York Medical College. As a recipient of a fellowship from the New York Heart Association, I had worked at the laboratory of Columbia University's Nobel Prize winner Dr. André Cournand, where I began research into human blood volume measurement. Along with Dr. Yale Enson, I discovered the first accurate method for gauging how much blood an individual has in his body, providing a high degree of accuracy not achievable previously.

In the course of my research, I had also developed emergency laboratory systems and often found my services requested by companies developing new products for the health care field. In 1974, I was asked to consult for a company called Idant, which was founded in 1971 to provide frozen semen for artificial insemination. This pioneering company was practically bankrupt and its technological premise—that it is possible to freeze and preserve human semen for years—was regarded with disbelief. Physicians at the time said that frozen semen was unnecessary, did not work, and was far inferior to fresh semen—despite the fact that fresh semen could not be tested for infectious agents prior to use.

Although I worked in the laboratory primarily on cardiac problems, I was originally trained in endocrinology, a field that encompasses fertility problems. I became convinced that freezing human semen was truly a unique advance in the treatment of male infertility. By matching the sperm donor to a husband's characteristics—with regard to race, ethnic background, height, weight, hair and eye color, blood group and type—it would now be possible for an infertile man to have a child by a genetically similar donor with respect to the above characteristics. The sperm from a semen donor could be cultured to make sure it was bacteria free, and the donor extensively tested prior to use of the semen. In addition, men undergoing chemotherapy for treatable cancers that would leave them sterile could now actually store their semen and have children at a later date.

Against the prevailing view that such a concept was doomed to failure, I joined my private scientific services consulting company to this pioneering cryobiology* laboratory and accepted the post of medical director of a new, combined corporation called Daxor, which included the Idant sperm bank. Within a year, some of the technical problems plaguing the process of freezing human semen and shipping it to doctors across the country were solved. Most of the other dozen human sperm banks started at this time went bankrupt but, despite several difficult years, Idant managed to survive, and frozen semen slowly began to gain acceptance as the best possible treatment for male sterility.

Acceptance was not immediate, however, and a majority of physicians continued to use fresh, untested semen. It was not until 1988, 14 years later, in the wake of AIDS, that the American Fertility Society and the federal Centers for Disease Control finally and officially stated that frozen semen and not fresh semen should be used for artificial insemination. It was a gratifying, if somewhat belated, recognition that only frozen, extensively tested semen was safe for artificial human insemination. By this time, Idant, the first public frozen sperm bank in the United States (and in the world), had also become the world's largest public frozen sperm bank, responsible for an estimated 15,000 births.

Soon after my involvement with Idant, it became apparent to me that if human sperm could be stored almost indefinitely at superlow temperatures, it should also be possible to store blood for prolonged periods of time. Pioneering researchers like Drs. Charles Huggins, Arthur Rowe, and Edmund Valeri had already proved that blood could be safely stored for several years in a frozen state. It occurred to me that just as individuals could store their own sperm for later use, it should be possible to store one's own blood for future use.

Almost immediately I began to investigate and test the feasibility of storing one's own blood as a practical matter. I soon discovered that the public at large, as well as most physicians, mistakenly thought that the available blood supply was quite safe. It became clear that the practice of storing blood for future use, especially if one had to pay for it, was a service very few people would utilize. Since sperm banking was not to gain acceptance for another five years, the concept of storing blood had to be shelved.

In 1985, an underwriter named D. H. Blair raised significant sums of money for the development of a blood-volume analyzer, an instrument designed by me on the basis of my years of research in human blood-volume measurement. That same year, with the death of movie

---

*Cryobiology is the science of freezing cells and tissue for long-term preservation.

star Rock Hudson from AIDS, the American public first became aware in a significant way that a new epidemic was threatening the country. By focusing attention on the mechanism of AIDS transmission, Hudson's death made clear that the epidemic was transmitted by a virus that could spread through the blood supply. Even beyond AIDS, the American people began to understand that blood transfusions were inherently dangerous, and autologous* donation—self-storage of blood—first received public notice. It appeared that the only safe blood was blood donated by an individual to himself, since this eliminated the danger of AIDS, hepatitis, or any transfusion reaction while guaranteeing a perfect match in blood types.

Repeated surveys during the eighties continued to show that a program for storing one's own blood would not be financially viable nor self-sustaining for many years, just as sperm-banking required years to become self-sustaining. I was also aware of repeated misleading asurances by most members of the blood banking establishment about the safety of the blood supply. It was clear that I would be subject to severe personal attacks were I to challenge the accepted wisdom and the power of this establishment. I had no illusions about the depth of the probable opposition, nor any doubt that the suggested reforms would be characterized as opportunistic in the face of public fears about the spreading AIDS epidemic. As this book will make abundantly clear, however, even if there were no AIDS epidemic, the blood banking system should have been reformed years before.

Despite these obstacles, in 1985 I elected to use a portion of the underwriting funds from my blood-volume analyzer to inaugurate the world's first public autologous blood bank—a respository where individuals could store blood for their own use or for the use of anyone else whom they might designate. It seems incredible that the obvious, inherent superiority of self-donated blood was not publicly acknowledged until 1986 by most segments of the medical and blood banking establishment. Just as there are now over 15,000 living children conceived from semen stored at Idant who would otherwise not have been born, as well as thousands of other children born from semen stored at other banks inspired by Idant's pioneering example, it was clear to me that a historic opportunity was at hand to provide a major advance in human blood transfusion technology.

Wartime sometimes stimulates research that has peacetime uses and saves thousands of lives; similarly, the AIDS crisis, by focusing

*Autologous means related to self, belonging to the same organism.

attention on the blood banking system, might serve as the catalyst
needed for the transition to a safe blood banking system. The opportunity to put into practice a program that could save thousands of
lives and improve the health of hundreds of thousands of people
comes to very few physcians in a lifetime. Accomplishing this would
also enable me to redeem the promise I had made years earlier.

For the record, I would also like to state that to date neither I nor
the company with which I am affiliated has made any profit from
blood banking. In fact, we have subsidized our blood service at an
extensive cost since its inception five years ago (meanwhile 19 other
companies who entered the field have either gone bankrupt or out of
business). From the beginning, we were aware that our blood service
would not be profitable for a long time, but we agreed to subsidize it
indefinitely because we believed it was a vital innovation whose time
would come.

In this book I have tried to outline some of the safe alternatives that
an informed public must choose if it wishes to protect itself from
current unsafe blood banking practices. In taking a voyage through
the history of the American blood banking system and exposing
many of the hidden flaws that still exist today, *Safe Blood* will have
some unsettling, even shocking things to say. For all our effort at
rational, scientific discussion, human blood is a symbolic, emotion-
ally charged subject. We are all aware from early childhood that blood
is essential to life. The sight of its fresh brilliant red color has such a
powerful effect that many people will faint at the sight of blood—particularly their own. In many primitive religions—and even among
some tribes today—man has practiced the ritual of drinking blood
from animals or humans. Universally, the shedding of blood has long
been a symbol of death.

Given this powerful cluster of associations, we do not like to hear
bad news about blood—or about the organizations responsible for
safeguarding the nation's blood supply, which we prefer to think of as
altruistic, charitable public servants. Unfortunately, this convenient
mythology has long masked many other realities. Today, with the
discovery of a host of life-threatening viruses—including, but in no
way confined to, the AIDS virus—we can no longer afford to ignore
the unnecessary dangers of our blood transfusion system or the fail-
ings of our blood banking organizations:

- Despite repeated assertions to the contrary, the current blood
  supply in the United States is unacceptably dangerous. The

risk of contracting AIDS from a blood transfusion is significantly higher than the public has been led to believe.

- The risk of transfusion hepatitis, and cirrhosis of the liver from hepatitis leading to death, is even higher than the risk of contracting AIDS.

- Blood is a multibillion dollar business and, contrary to their reputations, blood banking organizations do not always serve the best interests of American health, sometimes behaving more like business corporations than charities.*

- Today, the blood banking establishment employs a double standard in dealing with the dangers of the blood supply. The public at large is reassured that blood is safe, while special precautions are taken for selected groups (to be discussed in the following chapters), leaving the bulk of the 4 million Americans who receive a blood transfusion each year without necessary, additional safeguards that could be immediately implemented.

- The knowledge and the technology already exist for a safe blood banking system for all Americans.

In February 1988, on his 81st birthday, against all medical advice, my father went skiing. He took with him his 76-year-old brother-in-law, a physician who had previously undergone cardiac bypass surgery. To my father and uncle, skiing down a snowy slope was a celebration of life and their own indomitability.

In June 1988, my father developed chest pains and was rushed to Montefiore Hospital in the middle of the night. He was found to be anemic and received two units of blood donated by me, one fresh unit and one that I had previously frozen.

What originally appeared to be a heart attack turned out to be heart pain due to inadequate blood levels in the body. Further tests revealed a combination of cirrhosis of the liver and a possible tumor.

*As this book was being prepared for publication, Gilbert Gaul, a reporter for the *Philadelphia Inquirer,* won the Pulitzer Prize for his exposé of the blood industry, "The Blood Brokers." Gaul's series of articles led a congressional panel to open a wide-ranging investigation into the Food and Drug Administration's oversight of the blood industry. The House Energy and Commerce Subcommittee on Oversight and Investigations is looking at whether the FDA has the staff and the independence to regulate the billion-dollar industry, especially in the light of recent blood-safety problems.

Eight years earlier, when part of his colon was removed for cancer, my father had developed hepatitis from a transfusion. Now, the consulting hematologist told me that the liver-destroying cirrhosis caused by his previous hepatitis was my father's main medical problem.

Over the next three months my father was to receive more transfusions from me and my children. Liver failure from his chronic hepatitis reduced him to 104 pounds, unable to stand but completely lucid to the end. Like most people who develop hepatitis from a transfusion, my father was unaware in 1980 that he had contracted the disease, because it is apparent only if the appropriate liver tests are performed. It was only after my father became hopelessly ill that I informed him of his hepatitis as it is basically untreatable and I did not wish to worry him needlessly. Yet as I watched him wasting away in the final stages of his illness, I knew that he was dying from a disease that might have been avoided had safe blood been available. Four days after formally blessing his three grandsons, he expired, saying that he had made his peace with God and was prepared to leave.

In the fall of 1988, my 76-year-old physician uncle, a general practitioner who had won the 1944 Gold Medal from the Welcome Foundation (for the best research done in the military), suffered a stroke. In February 1989, he announced to his thousands of patients in Pittsfield, Massachusetts that after 50 years, the time had come for him to give up the practice of medicine.

This book is dedicated to my uncle, Dr. Carl Wildman, who was my inspiration to become a physician; and to my father, Carl Feldschuh, a man of courage whose personal experience with transfusion was a constant spur to develop a system that I strongly hope will save many lives.

———

Doron Weber wishes to acknowledge Dr. Joseph Feldschuh for the steadfastness, vision, and enterprise of the genuine reformer; Erwin Glikes for his solid commitment and intelligent stewardship of the book; Adam Bellow for his fine, skillful editing and his friendship; Edith Lewis for her patient guidance through the indispensable tasks of editorial production; also Renata and Nancy and the entire gang at the Writers Room in New York, for the space and support to write; and a special acknowledgment of gratitude and love to Shealagh, my wife, and Damon, my son.

1

A Dangerous
Misunderstanding

Does this mean that all is now well and that the future safety of the
blood supply is assured? We don't think so. First, we are distressed
that so many blood bankers and organizations still do not understand
that more could have been done from 1983–5 to prevent
transfusion-associated AIDS. This suggests that they simply don't
realize that the system failed or that it has flaws.

> *Dr. Edgar G. Engleman, Stanford University Blood Center, before the*
> *Presidential Commission on the HIV Epidemic, May 1988*

American public health is lower than necessary because the quality of
our blood is lower than necessary.

> *Professor Ross Eckert, member of FDA Blood Products Advisory Committee,*
> Statement on Blood Safety, *May 1988*

In the United States right now, someone needs a blood transfusion
every 3.75 seconds.[1] Before the year is out, this will add up to 4
million newly transfused Americans. There is a high statistical proba-
bility that you—whoever you are and whatever you do—will require
at least one transfusion of blood by the time you are 72. Indeed, some
estimates claim that there is a 95 percent chance that you will require
either a blood transfusion or a blood product at some point in your
lifetime.[2]

Blood transfusions often begin with birth, as a vital aid to obstetric
care—and they may be the last form of therapy for patients on a

hospital deathbed. From cradle to grave, blood transfusions affect our lives.

Blood is the most precious fluid on earth, yet it can also be one of the most toxic. Of the 4 million Americans who received blood last year, between 200,000 and 400,000—or at least 500 people a day— will contract hepatitis alone.[3] Thousands of these will eventually die from cirrhosis of the liver. Disease-causing viruses such as cytomega- lovirus (CMV), Epstein-Barr virus, HTLV-I, HTLV-II, HIV-2, and dis- eases such as malaria, Lyme disease, Chagas' disease, and occasionally even syphilis, as well as other diseases, will continue to spread through the blood supply and infect increasing numbers of transfu- sion recipients. Perhaps most alarming of all, in 1990 the risk of contracting AIDS from a blood transfusion is significantly higher than the public perceives. While most attention has focused on those who contracted acquired immune deficiency syndrome, or AIDS, from a blood transfusion before mandatory AIDS testing was initi- ated in 1985—12,000 to 15,000 transfusion recipients are known to have been infected before 1985,[4] plus an additional 10,000 hemophil- iacs[5]—the safety of the American blood supply today is still danger- ously compromised by the presence of the AIDS virus. While no one knows exactly how widespread the danger is, estimates are signifi- cantly higher than we have been led to believe. For example:

- Based on figures from the Centers for Disease Control (CDC), we may conclude that as many as 1 in 7,400 patients nationwide who receive transfusions will contract AIDS from tainted blood.[6]*
- Based on CDC figures, in New York and other high-risk urban centers, the risk of AIDS could be five to ten times higher than in the rest of the country, which suggests that anywhere from 1 in 750 to 1 in 1,500 patients receiving blood transfusions may contract AIDS from contaminated blood.

Given these risks, is our society now getting the safest available blood for transfusion? The answer is no. Do safer alternatives exist? The answer is yes.

Of course, any medical procedure involves a certain element of risk, and doctors are generally willing to accept a degree of mortality as long as the overall results are beneficial. Absolute safety or perfec- tion is not attainable and can never be guaranteed for blood transfu-

*For an explanation of these figures, see note 6 (p. 182) and Chap. 6.

sions or for any other major therapeutic procedure. However, this qualification can itself become an excuse for not doing all that we can. When it comes to transfusion therapy today, there are several known, well-documented improvements which could go far toward reducing the high rate of infection in the blood supply, but these precautions are being resisted by an entrenched and powerful bureaucracy. The result is that the majority of the 4 million blood recipients in the United States are placed in unnecessary danger each year and prevented from making their own decisions about the best available treatment for them.

Unfortunately, the blood banking establishment employs a double standard in dealing with the known dangers of the blood supply. The public at large is assured that blood is safe, while special precautions are taken for selected groups. For example, according to a 1988 FDA recommendation, certain groups of paid plasma donors who receive small transfusions in order to form antibody-rich blood are now granted special safeguards.[7] These privileged donors will receive only frozen blood that has been quarantined and retested after six months. Blood bankers believe that only in this way can the danger of AIDS, where detectable antibodies may not form for several months or more, be effectively eliminated. However, the 4 million Americans who receive blood transfusions each year—and who face the same hazards from the general blood supply—do not receive the same protection. They are transfused with blood that has not been quarantined and retested, placing them at significantly increased risk.

One of the bitter ironies of the growing AIDS crisis is that even these extra precautions for select groups may turn out to be inadequate. On June 1, 1989, the *New England Journal of Medicine* published a major new study suggesting that infection with the AIDS virus may be undetectable for *three years or more* despite the use of the current AIDS antibody test.[8] Of 31 homosexual men infected with AIDS in this study, only 4 tested positive on the standard AIDS antibody test within three years. In other words, for every AIDS carrier detected within the three-year period, there were seven undetectable carriers. This strongly suggests that even a six-month quarantine period—during which one waits for AIDS antibodies to show up—is inadequate for satisfactory protection. According to these findings, to ensure that the blood supply is free of AIDS, one might theoretically have to wait more than three years to see if AIDS antibodies have developed in donor blood.

A similar double standard exists with respect to blood tests and artificial insemination. In February 1988, the FDA recommended that only frozen sperm be used for artificial insemination: in this way sperm donors have their blood tested at the time of sperm donation, and then six months later, before their quarantined sperm can be released for use.[9] Again, regulatory authorities believe that this is the only sure way to guard against the transmission of AIDS. The result is that women receiving sperm from semen donors are granted additional safeguards against known risks while the general public remains uninformed about such risks.[10]

The current blood banking system in the United States is inadequate and seriously flawed. Despite some genuine improvements, the blood we get in our hospitals for transfusion today is not as safe as it should and could be; and despite public assurances, many of us are still paying for this deficiency with our lives. This book will explain what is wrong with blood banking and transfusion practice today, how and why the system developed into its present organizational form, and what steps our society can take to remedy this dangerous situation. It will also suggest what individuals can do immediately to protect themselves and their families from a blood banking establishment that has yet to make their best interest its first priority.

Part of the current problem lies with the ruling powers of the American blood banking establishment. The industry that is responsible for collecting whole blood in the United States and supplying it to hospitals has functioned largely as a privileged cartel.

Dominated by the colossus of the American Red Cross and a trade group known as the American Association of Blood Banks (AABB), the industry has been largely protected from legitimate competition by various regulatory policies. Mishandling of the blood supply has been shielded by laws limiting legal liability and hence any genuine accountability. The federal regulator, the FDA, acts at times more like an advocate than an overseer; its members are closely allied with blood banking interests and, according to the Presidential Commission on the HIV Epidemic, "It relies heavily on that industry for advice on what standards to set—a relationship that presents a significant opportunity for conflicts of interest to arise."[11] Meanwhile, the industry's official status as a "not-for-profit" enterprise has at times lent it a spurious moral authority while making it exempt from paying taxes.

This "not-for-profit" status is deceptive, since the whole blood industry reaps tremendous profits from blood banking, a business whose sales exceed $1 billion a year.[12] The Red Cross, without surrendering any of its exemptions, even competes in the plasma sector, the other half of the blood industry which is dominated by large commercial manufacturers on an avowedly for-profit basis. The sale of plasma—the yellowish, liquid part of the blood which is manufactured into special products for hemophiliacs, shock and burn victims and others—also accounts for well over a billion dollars in revenues each year.[13]

The Red Cross Blood Services has annual revenues of over half a billion dollars and a percentage of profits that would place it near the top of the Fortune 500.[14] Because of its supposedly altruistic mission, its long and impressive record of service in other fields, and its special charter as a quasi-government agency, few have been willing to challenge this revered institution.

Nevertheless, the Red Cross Blood Services has at times behaved in a self-serving commercial manner that is at odds with the best interest of public health—and with its own official status as a charitable institution. Although the American Red Cross performs numerous other public services, its lucrative Blood Services division alone accounts for 60 percent of its total revenues.[15] It is hardly surprising, then, that the Red Cross has invested so much effort in protecting its economic lifeblood.

One of the popular myths disseminated by the Red Cross is that its blood is free, a claim that is misleading. The Red Cross, the AABB, and a third group known as the Council of Community Blood Banks (CBCC) do collect free blood from volunteers; but they then sell that blood to hospitals at a profit. Strictly speaking, of course, they are not selling the blood "product" but the "service" of collecting, storing, processing and distributing blood to hospitals. Only in this limited sense can the Red Cross maintain that it provides "free" blood to everyone. The actual charge, called a "cost-recovery fee," is usually well above cost.

One unit of whole blood collected from a volunteer is commonly broken down into several components—red cells, platelets, plasma—and each component is then sold separately to hospitals for a higher total than the original unit would bring on its own. All these costs are passed on to patients with substantial hospital mark-ups. A pint of blood given for free by a donor can become a $600 product by the time it reaches the consumer.

In another inconsistency, the nominally "non-profit" Red Cross also generates revenues of over $80 million a year by selling plasma derivatives in the commercial "for-profit" sector.[16] In this enterprise the Red Cross Blood Services has many advantages over for-profit pharmaceutical companies: its raw material or plasma is free, since it does not pay its donors; its advertising is free, saving millions of dollars a year; a significant part of its labor is free, since it is composed of volunteers; and it is completely tax exempt.[17]

For years, pharmaceutical companies have been complaining about unfair competition and clamoring for redress. At the present time Congress is reexamining some of these Red Cross privileges as part of a larger investigation of "commercial and other income-producing activities of organizations that have tax-exempt status under Section 501 of the Internal Revenue Code."[18]

Commercial manufacturers like Alpha Therapeutics have testified that the Red Cross Blood Services Division is "abusing" its tax exempt status and competing "unfairly" with private enterprise in an activity that has "no substantial relationship to the organization's exempt purpose."[19] The Red Cross Blood Services may not be alone in taking advantage of federal tax laws, but since it deals in public health—and appeals to public trust—its putative violations may have far-reaching consequences.

"Nonprofit" organizations rely on other useful myths as well. For example, the Red Cross has historically opposed commercial or paid blood as "bad" and voluntary blood as "good," creating an artificial but powerful moral distinction. In practice, the distinction between voluntary nonprofit blood banks and commercial for-profit companies is far from clear or simple. While paid donors have been and are currently associated with higher rates of hepatitis—especially poor or derelict donors who lie about their health in order to get $10 or $15 for their blood—not all paid donors are bad. In fact, several studies in the seventies, including one at the Mayo Clinic, showed that when registries are maintained, paid donors may actually be safer than voluntary donors. But the distinction has stuck and, widely publicized by an influential book called *The Gift Relationship* (published in 1972),[20] and supported by a National Blood Policy enacted in 1974, it resulted in the stigmatization of commercial blood banks and the increasing dominance or regionalization of the nation's blood supply by nonprofit collectors.

It was not until the advent of the AIDS epidemic that the claims of nonprofit organizations to be the best and safest suppliers of the nation's blood were openly challenged. After it was identified in 1981, AIDS quickly became the nation's number one health concern. When, in late 1982, the CDC (federal Centers for Disease Control) announced that AIDS was caused by a virus that could be transmitted through the blood, AIDS also became the nation's newest transfusion threat.[21] However, the organizations entrusted with supplying the nation's transfusion blood—primarily the American Red Cross and most members of the American Association of Blood Banks—failed to provide adequate and timely protection against this new threat.[22]

In criticizing the response to AIDS, and many policies of the Red Cross and the AABB, an important distinction must be made between the many dedicated, able professionals within these organizations who try to serve the public's best interest* and the organizations' actions as powerful institutions protecting their vested interests. One of our chief areas of contention concerns the emergence of blood banking as a multibillion-dollar industry where corporate concerns influence and may even override sound medical decisions.

To date between 200 and 300 lawsuits are still pending against blood banks across the nation.[23] The lawsuits allege that blood banks were negligent in their efforts to keep the AIDS virus out of the blood supply before the introduction of an AIDS-antibody screening test in mid-1985. While plaintiffs have apparently won three of the five cases that reached a jury trial, two of the three are being appealed by the blood banks that lost. Based on previous decisions, there is a good chance of reversal. The third case, which the blood bank clearly lost, has been settled out of court for an undisclosed sum. Like the tobacco industry, which has yet to admit that cigarette smoking can cause cancer, blood banks consistently deny any culpability for fear of establishing a legal precedent. Yet their long delay and inaction before mid-1985 certainly contributed to many tragedies. Some independent blood bankers and concerned physicians have called for a formal inquiry into the industry's performance between 1983 and 1985.[24] Ironically, the blood banks' continued denial of the current risks may be laying the groundwork for lawsuits in the mid-nineties.

In Florida, a father was prevented from giving blood to his own son after an auto accident.[25] The boy was forced to accept random blood for his transfusion—blood from an anonymous donor pool—despite the fact that 5 to 10 percent of transfusion recipients contract an infection after a blood transfusion. In court the judge upheld the blood bank since their decision was in keeping with standard operating procedure in the industry. Although in this much-publicized case the boy did not become ill from his transfusion, many members of the public were shocked that a blood bank could legally prevent a father from donating blood to his own son.

Other patients who tried to predonate their own blood for surgery or to store it for some future contingency also were met with many

*The author is himself a member of the AABB.

bureaucratic obstacles and strong opposition—and with still more dire consequences. In New Jersey, a man facing elective surgery was prevented from predonating his own blood and from designating friends and family to donate blood for him. The hospital argued that they did not accept this form of personal donation, which they considered selfish and mean-spirited. Compelled to receive anonymous blood from the general blood supply, the man eventually developed AIDS as a result of his transfusion. He is now suing the hospital and the blood bank.[26]

In California, a baby boy born prematurely was in dire need of transfusions. The infant's father requested that he and other family members be allowed to donate blood for the baby. According to court documents, despite bitter protests the resident physician refused the family's request, stating that directed donations were against hospital policy. Despite his parents' express wishes, the newborn child received 22 separate components of blood from the general supply before he left the hospital. The blood was contaminated with AIDS and the boy developed a full-blown case of the disease. He is now on the drug AZT, but his family failed in their lawsuit against the hospital.[27]

These cases, and hundreds like them, demonstrate that when it comes to the strange laws governing blood, individual citizens appear not to have full rights to choose their own treatment or to avoid preventable risks they do not wish to take.

To appreciate the injustice of such a policy, it is useful to understand that *a blood transfusion is the most intimate contact you can have with another human being. It is more intimate than sex.* Medically speaking, a blood transfusion is equivalent to a transplant. A part of someone else's body is removed and placed into the body of a patient. In any free country, one can choose one's own sexual partner through mutual consent. Yet under current blood banking policy in many hospitals and localities, one is forced into the most intimate contact with a total stranger. The organizations responsible for this policy assert that it is done for the patient's own good, an arguable claim at best. Yet as will be shown, these same organizations, whom we trust with this responsibility, do not always avail themselves of the many possibilities that exist to increase the safety of a transfusion. Fortunately this policy is beginning to crumble under pressure from a gradually awakening public, who wish to take a more active role and assume more responsibility for vital decisions that are being made on their behalf.

Since nonprofit organizations do not pay their donors, they must rely on altruism and good will. These are not always the strongest motivators. Blood bankers, therefore, must constantly expand their recruitment efforts, sometimes casting their net too widely or indiscriminately in an effort to keep up with the demand for blood. As AIDS began to spread in the 1980s, the Red Cross and the AABB faced a serious, potential loss of donors.

A blood banker's greatest fear is always a shortage of donors. While he has a legitimate right to be concerned about losing donors, his first concern and top priority must always be the safety of the blood supply. Yet when the CDC first announced that AIDS could be transmitted through blood, the Red Cross and the AABB avoided the adoption of rigorous screening procedures for fear of offending the sensibilities of certain high-risk groups and of discouraging new donors by tough, intrusive questioning.[28]

An additional concern was that potential loss of donors could lead to a loss of revenues and possible staff layoffs for blood banks.[29] Blood shortages in turn might lead hospitals to look elsewhere, or to form their own blood banks.

Such behavior contrasted, in the mid-eighties, with that of commercial plasma collectors, who did take greater precautions to protect their clients from the risk of AIDS by initiating additional screening procedures to protect the source of supply and by reducing the frequency of potentially high-risk donors two years earlier. In this case, for-profit companies outperformed "nonprofit" organizations in their efforts to protect the blood supply.

Compounding this early reticence, for two critical years when there was no direct test for AIDS antibodies, the Red Cross, the AABB, and the CCBC leadership refused to accept any surrogate or substitute test such as the T-cell test and the hepatitis B core antibody test to screen blood for AIDS. Meanwhile several independent blood bankers across the country were doing this with some success.[30] Since these surrogate tests were not specific—AIDS could not yet be tested directly—their adoption would have forced blood collectors to throw out some good blood along with the contaminated specimens.

While some individual blood bankers performed extra tests as AIDS spread through the national blood supply, the Red Cross and the AABB did not initiate any additional tests or procedures that might have lowered the number of people eventually infected with the disease. During this period, over 11 million units of blood were collected and more than 15 million units distributed to hospitals.[31] We may never know how many thousands of people were unnecessarily infected as a result of this delay. Current estimates are that 25,000 Americans, including 10,000 hemophiliacs, contracted AIDS from a blood transfusion before 1985.[32]

Today the result is a serious crisis of confidence in the use of transfusions. Blood banking organizations counter that these fears are unwarranted and that the blood supply is safer than ever. It is true that, in response to growing publicity about AIDS and widespread criticism about their performance, blood bankers have taken some steps to improve the supply. Two new tests have been adopted for hepatitis, the hepatitis B core antibody test and ALT liver enzyme test.* These tests had been recommended for years and consistently rejected by the blood banking establishment.[33] (One of them, the core antibody test, was initially rejected by the Red Cross and the AABB as a surrogate test for AIDS.) Though too late in coming, these tests have somewhat reduced the risk of hepatitis in the blood supply.

To its credit, the Red Cross has been more aggressive in testing for HTLV-I, a new cancer-causing AIDS-related virus that has been spreading dangerously. And it has also begun to offer some limited patient-directed and autologous (self-donated) blood transfusion programs. Yet serious doubts persist about whether there has been any fundamental change in the industry.

Dr. Edgar Engleman, the Stanford blood bank director who became something of a national figure when he began surrogate testing two years before the Red Cross, reads an ominous signal in the industry's inability to admit its previous failures and the system's general malfunctioning. Engleman claims that there has still not been any internal investigation by blood-banking organizations into what went wrong. Rather, these organizations have maintained an Olympian impassivity, admitting only what is simply undeniable. Testifying before the Presidential Commission on AIDS in May 1988, Engleman called for a formal inquiry into the industry's performance:

"The recent adoption of stringent new blood testing procedures may possibly represent a response to public pressure rather than a result of self-examination. When the current public outcry abates, can we be confident that the industry will respond to future unforeseen problems?"[34]

Given the blood industry's record, this is a valid and disturbing question. Yet even with the present, already known problems, the industry is still not doing enough. Not only does the blood supply

*ALT is the enzyme alanine aminotransferase. This enzyme circulates in large amounts through the blood when the liver has been damaged, as in hepatitis. The hepatitis B core antibody test detects antibodies at the core of the hepatitis B virus and thus indicates past exposure to hepatitis B.

system today remain too dangerous but the blood industry persists in denying the significance of that danger, especially when one considers the steps that could be taken to lower the risk from a transfusion.

AIDS continues to be a potential threat for every transfusion recipient. There is still no practical, economical, direct test for the presence of the AIDS virus in the blood.[35] The present test can only detect the presence of antibodies that form in response to infection with the AIDS virus. Since there may be a lag of three months to three years or even more between infection with the AIDS virus and the appearance of AIDS antibodies, an unknown quantity of AIDS-tainted blood is still slipping through this "window" and infecting the blood supply.

Some patients may take at least 35 months to produce AIDS antibodies.[36] Recent findings also suggest that the virus can conceal itself in specialized immune-system cells called macrophages without triggering any antibodies at all—and so remain permanently undetectable by the present test.[37] The most accurate test for detection of early AIDS is a DNA PCR test, a very difficult and expensive test to perform which is capable of detecting the AIDS virus months or years before the antibody test turns positive.

Some AIDS high-risk donors are still not being adequately screened and deterred from donating blood. Before testing donated blood for AIDS, the first and obvious line of defense is to ask those at high risk for the disease to exclude themselves as donors. However, in practice this does not always work.[38] Today high-risk individuals continue to donate blood. Many of these are inadvertent carriers who do not know they are infected. Some are known high-risk candidates who are ill-informed; others feel socially pressured to donate; some use the opportunity to get a free AIDS test. Without doubt, the current practice of relying on personal discretion—on donor self-exclusion—is dangerously limited.

Finally, there are critics who continue to question the effectiveness of screening for any single virus with HIV.[39] The genetic structure of the AIDS virus is so highly variable—with seven isolates known already—that it may be futile to single out and test for only one virus.

The best medical estimate today is that we are at least 10 to 20 years from developing an AIDS vaccine. Yet even if a cure for AIDS were discovered tomorrow, the blood supply would still not be safe.

The biggest threat of all is hepatitis, which has been very conservatively estimated to kill 4,000 transfusion recipients a year.[40] Between 1 in 10 and 1 in 15 transfusion recipients will contract hepatitis. The vast majority of these cases involve hepatitis non-A non-B. That adds

up to over 200,000 potential hepatitis victims every year—and possibly as many as 400,000. A recent test under development claims to
eliminate many of these cases. But while one hopes for the best—and
though preliminary results are promising—it is important to note
that similar claims were made 15 years ago, when hepatitis B was
thought to be the last threat to the blood supply. One of the problems
is that the new test only detects a single hepatitis virus, called hepatitis
C, whereas hepatitis is believed to be caused by multiple, unidentified
viruses. It will take many years before we can determine the effectiveness of this new test, which is just now being introduced. The hepatitis
B test took seven years to evaluate. In the meantime, hepatitis remains
a very serious risk for any patient in need of a blood transfusion.

New viruses from the AIDS family of retroviruses, HIV-2, HTLV-I
and HTLV-II, pose a growing danger to the blood supply. A new test
for HTLV-I has been adopted but, as with the test for AIDS, questions
persist about a window period for this elusive retrovirus. Disease-
causing viruses like CMV and Epstein-Barr virus, and diseases such as
malaria, Lyme disease, Chagas' disease, and syphilis, are all transmissible through the blood. Even more disturbing are new mutations of
existing viruses that are not detectable by the current tests. The blood
supply remains an open conduit for dangerous microorganisms. Nor
can we ever be sure what the newest virus or mutation will be.

Aware of these risks, researchers are constantly searching for alternatives to transfusion. Artificial blood has been talked about for 25
years but no one has yet succeeded in creating a safe, effective blood
substitute. The synthetic blood that was made from fluorocarbons in
the 1970s has not fulfilled its expectations. More recently, artificial
hemoglobin from discarded human blood has shown some promise,
but it is too toxic and short-lived. Despite ongoing efforts, artificial
blood remains a far-off goal and not a realistic alternative to human
blood today.

Blood cleansing, the process of sterilizing blood of its contaminants, has also attracted scientists. Complex heating techniques are
presently employed with some success to deactivate viruses from
certain plasma products. Whole blood and its components have
proved more problematic because it is impossible at the present time
kill off all infectious agents without damaging the rest of the blood.
The latest experimental techniques involve the use of laser beams and
chemical dyes. While still in their preliminary stages, these methods
have not yet proven safe or effective as a means of cleansing blood of
its viral contaminants.

Today there does exist a better alternative to receiving blood at random from a huge, anonymous donor pool that is inadequately screened and tested. The alternative is to use your own blood. No other blood is as safe for the patient as his or her own. The risk of infection or of any kind of transfusion reaction is virtually eliminated. Today there is near unanimity that "the safest blood is your own"—although it was not until 1986 that organizations like the American Red Cross, the National Institutes of Health, the American Medical Association, and the FDA made an effort to acknowledge this self-evident concept publicly.

The process of donating blood to oneself is known as autologous transfusion as opposed to homologous transfusion, where the blood comes from another donor. With the AIDS scare, self-storage of blood has begun to be accepted by the public. Autologous donation is growing in popularity, having doubled in each of the last two years so that it now accounts for almost 5 percent of all blood donated.[41] After years of strewing objections in its path, the American Red Cross and the AABB have begun to support this practice in a limited fashion.

However, as will be explained in later chapters, the form of autologous donation encouraged today by the Red Cross and the AABB—namely, predonation prior to surgery—is seriously flawed. In the first place, at best only 10 percent of transfusion recipients are eligible for this form of self-donation and the real figure is probably closer to 5 percent.[42] Under presurgical blood donation, the patient comes in each week before his operation and donates a pint of blood. The result is that he enters surgery—just when he most needs his strength—in an anemic and blood-depleted state. It is potentially a very dangerous practice to bleed down and weaken patients, many of them elderly and already feeble, on the eve of a major operation.

Current FDA guidelines stipulate that a *healthy* person must not donate more than once every 8 weeks in order to regain his normal blood volume.* Yet a sick person in need of surgery is now supposedly safe to donate up to two pints of blood in one week. It is difficult for any concerned medical practitioner to justify such a dangerous approach when safer solutions are readily available.

In fact, autologous transfusion as practiced today may be *more* dangerous than receiving blood at random from a complete stranger. Taking multiple units of blood from a patient just prior to surgery is really a stop-gap measure used to counter the growing fear of transfusion-AIDS. But by leaving the patient weak and anemic, such blood depletion may do more harm than good, since to operate on a person

*This 8-week exclusion can be waived at the discretion of the blood bank director.

who has lost two to three pints of blood in a few weeks exposes that individual to an increased risk of a stroke or heart attack.

Another growing danger of the AIDS-induced fear of transfusion is the practice of *undertransfusion*. Many doctors would rather risk operating on a patient with thinned-out blood—holding off on a transfusion—than expose that patient to AIDS. And many worried patients are themselves refusing transfusions. The NIH (National Institutes of Health), along with scores of other medical groups, has recommended that ordinary homologous transfusions (blood from other donors) be "reduced to a minimum."[43]

Most doctors are now permitting patients to bleed to ever-lower levels before they order a transfusion. Since they do not feel secure about the safety of the blood supply, doctors are reluctant to give adequate replacement. In this atmosphere of panic and uncertainty, patients are simply not getting enough blood. This leaves them vulnerable during any operation to blood-related complications such as stroke or heart attack; and even after an operation, many doctors continue to withhold blood out of the same anxiety. As a result, many patients suffer complications and some may even die unnecessarily.

It is impossible to measure the full extent of this dangerous practice, since the cause of death when patients die from undertransfusion is simply attributed to the underlying condition—the reason why the patient was hospitalized in the first place. It should not be surprising that most doctors refrain from volunteering that a patient died not from his original illness, but because his vital organs were starved of oxygen due to undertransfusion. Yet this happens with some frequency, and as a physician I have witnessed such cases myself. There have been cases wherein individuals unexpectedly died after relatively simple surgical procedures, such as gall bladder surgery, when no blood was given and death may have been caused by a similar fear of giving AIDS-contaminated blood. If doctors could feel confident about the safety of the blood supply, they would not hesitate to give patients adequate blood replacement and thus avoid many of these complications; and patients, with safe blood on hand, would not be denied its many therapeutic benefits.

There is one method to guarantee safe blood and that is to donate your own blood and freeze it until it is needed. Modern techniques of freezing allow for the safe storage of blood for up to 20 years. The FDA recently increased the official allowable period for frozen blood storage from 3 to 10 years. You cannot contract AIDS or hepatitis, or suffer any kind of transfusion reaction from your own blood. You do not have to deplete your own supply and weaken yourself prior to surgery if you have stored and frozen blood prior to any anticipated need. And no doctor will choose to withhold needed blood from you, or postpone surgery, when he has a safe quantity of your own blood in store.

Frozen, autologous donation allows people to take the personal initiative and responsibility to create their own private frozen blood banking supply. Ideally, all the members of a family can join the system and provide cross-coverage. So can close friends or other approved parties. When there is not enough of one's own blood for personal use, blood from pretested family members or friends can be far safer than blood from the general supply.

The Red Cross and the AABB oppose frozen autologous blood on the grounds that it will damage voluntary donation and create blood shortages. This view, which would be a source of genuine concern for the public if it were true, is not supported by the evidence. Only about 4 percent of the population now donates blood every year for the whole country, so there is a large, untapped pool of potential donors.[44] Autologous donation increases involvement by bringing more people into the blood bank who otherwise would never have donated. To the extent that people have their own supply of blood available, it also alleviates some of the pressure on organizations like the Red Cross to supply blood for the general population. Many people who cannot be blood donors for others—because of medication or infection—can still be donors for themselves. In addition, frozen, autologous blood that has been screened and tested and proven to be safe can obviously be used for individuals other than the original donor once he or she no longer needs the blood. In this way, frozen blood acts as an *additional* source of blood which can actually help to alleviate the frequent, severe donor blood shortages.

While the concept of freezing and storing one's own blood before it is needed is still relatively new, the idea has steadily been winning adherents. When Pope John Paul II met with Ronald Reagan in Miami in 1987, it was reported that both leaders were bringing their own personal blood supply with them as a precautionary measure.[45] A fully stocked rescue truck with a trauma team accompanied each man on his visit, carrying a ready supply of his own blood. Singer-celebrity Michael Jackson is also reputed to carry his own frozen blood with him wherever he goes.*

Frozen self-storage of blood, however, is not available only to the

---

*As will be shown later, in a well-designed system it is not necessary to travel with one's own blood.

powerful and wealthy. In 1987, Steve Ross, then president of Warner Communications, became the first head of a major corporation to offer this service to all his employees in the Unites States. Other companies have since followed suit, making frozen self-storage of blood a real option for increasing numbers of working Americans. Meanwhile the Japanese, who have high rates of hepatitis and other blood-borne diseases, have also shown great interest in this concept. In 1988, the AIM corporation, a privately held financial corporation of Japan, contracted with the Daxor Corporation, whose Idant division started the first public autologous blood bank in the United States, to help develop the first frozen autologous blood bank in Japan.

Clearly, the dangers and shortcomings that plague the blood supply and the blood transfusion system are a matter for global concern and cooperation. Not only did AIDS-contaminated blood infect 10,000 American hemophiliacs—or half the nation's hemophiliac population—by 1985, but the United States, the world's largest exporter of plasma, sent AIDS-contaminated blood to plasma importers such as Japan and West Germany.[46] In West Germany, one of America's biggest plasma customers, 3,000 of the country's 6,000 hemophiliacs have been infected with the AIDS virus.[47]

There are many objections to the use of frozen, autologous blood, and these will be dealt with in later chapters. One cannot underestimate the fierce opposition and criticism that such a program has met and may continue to meet in the near future. But medical science advances slowly, and the harbingers of change are rarely greeted with open arms. One hundred years ago, Ignaz Philipp Semmelweis, an Austrian physician, was ridiculed and ultimately forced to resign from his hospital position for daring to suggest that all medical personnel wash their hands before an operation. It was common practice in his day for doctors to go directly from the morgue, where they were performing autopsies on diseased bodies, to the hospital delivery room. Women in childbirth frequently contracted infections, and Semmelweis was the first physician to realize that the precaution of washing one's hands might reduce their incidence and spread.

Twenty-five years from now medical experts and historians may look back in disbelief at our practice of uncritically accepting blood from total strangers for transfusion into our veins when safer alternatives existed. It may seem inexplicable that we tolerated a 5 to 10 percent chance of infection and the very real risk of fatality when we had the technology to reduce this danger markedly.

Blood is a big business in America—over two billion dollars a year, expected almost to double by 1993—and there are powerful, vested interests who seek to perpetuate their control over it. Fortunately, the age of consumer awareness has caught up with blood banking; and recent public revelations have exposed some of the flaws in the current system. As people become better informed, they will demand better quality. At the very least, every citizen should know the full range of options and be entitled to make up his or her own mind. No one should be forced to accept anything less than the best health care available, and it is the purpose of this book to help individuals, should the need ever arise, to obtain the best blood available for themselves and their families. Every person should have the basic right to use his or her own blood when available or to select another specific blood donor if circumstances permit. No person should be compelled to accept anonymous blood from unknown donors or from donors who have been given only minimal standard tests when significantly improved testing methods and programs exist to lower the incidence of infection from transfusion. The public should never tolerate a policy that would take away the most basic right of a patient: the control of one's own body.

2

Transfusion History
and Practice

It took thousands of years to gain a rudimentary understanding of
how blood circulates through the body. Following this momentous
discovery by William Harvey in the seventeenth century, the first
efforts at transfusion involved injecting the blood of sheep or dogs
into the human circulatory system. As recently as the 1870s in New
York, cow's milk was enthusiastically championed as the magical
elixir for intravenous therapy. Thus for hundreds of years after an
understanding of the circulation, little progress was made despite
sporadic breakthroughs.

It is only in this century that the lifesaving capacities of blood have
been effectively understood and blood transfusions utilized as an
integral part of the health care system. The relatively late development of therapeutic blood transfusion makes a remarkable, ongoing
story. But the happy ending, as this book will try to show, has yet to be
written. Twenty-five years from now the present routine practice of
taking blood from a totally anonymous donor may come to seem as
scientifically primitive as previous transfusion experiments with milk
or sheep's blood seem to us today.

EARLY MYTHS AND THEORIES OF BLOOD

The idea that blood and life are closely linked is an ancient one—
nearly as old as the idea that it might be possible to sustain life by

19

transferring blood from one individual to another. For thousands of years, an almost mystical reverence attached to the alleged properties of this mysterious fluid.

Primitive peoples knew that an injury causing large blood loss resulted in death, or a loss of the spirit. Cave drawings at Altamira in Spain show that 30,000 years ago man recognized the presence of a vital fluid in the body: if you lost enough of it, you would die. A famous biblical injunction in Leviticus (17:11) also links blood directly with life: "Ye shall not eat the blood of no maner of flesh: for the life of all flesh is the blood thereof."* When Homer wished to describe a warrior bleeding to death, he referred to the "life spirit" that fled from his limbs.

Blood was associated with the essence of life itself, and people were eager to partake of all they could. The ancient Egyptians were known to use blood baths for refreshment and recuperation, much as we take spring or salt baths today. The Romans reputedly rushed into the arena to drink the blood of dying gladiators. They believed the spurting red fluid had a tonic effect and would rejuvenate them. Celsus, the great first-century medical writer, describes great Roman orgies of blood-guzzling as an aspect of the search for a fountain of youth.[1]

The first transfusions were really blood drafts—taken orally as opposed to injection—and could not have been very effective. In 1492, Pope Innocent VIII was reported to have received blood from three young men. He was in a coma and the blood, probably administered as a drink, did not help. The pontiff died, as did all three donors.[2]

The theory of the four humors, first propounded in the second century by the Greek physician Galen, dominated Western ideas about blood for 1,400 years.[3] At bottom, this doctrine expressed a belief in blood as one of the mystical products that embodied the physical and emotional characteristics of its owner. According to Galen's theory, there were four fundamental "humors" present in man: blood, phlegm, black bile, and yellow bile. Like the four elements, each of these humors corresponded to different physical states: "hot" for blood, "cold" for phlegm, "moist" for black bile, and "dry" for yellow bile.

For centuries, physicians believed that the measure of disease or health in an individual was a direct result of the equilibrium or

---

*Jehovah's Witnesses interpret this so strictly that today they still refuse lifesaving blood transfusions, even for their children.

imbalance among these humors. If blood predominated in your makeup, you were a ruddy, manic, "sanguine" type; if phlegm, you were pale, lackluster, and "phlegmatic"; black bile made you dark, angry, and "bilious"; and yellow bile indicated you were depressed or "melancholic." These adjectives still linger in our vocabulary today, showing the stubbornness of certain deeply embedded ideas. The long association of blood with inheritance is similarly revealed today in terms like "blue blood" and "bad blood."

The theory of the four humors implied that bad or discolored blood—a preponderance of one humor or shade over the others—was a cause rather than an effect of illness. From this erroneous premise, it was only a short jump to the practice of bloodletting: the draining off or purging of the offending humor until the patient regained a normal color and a "healthy" equilibrium.

Bloodletting was practiced freely and widely. It was a quick and simple procedure; a vein was punctured in the forearm and the blood let out. No physician was required; any barber-surgeon could perform this negative transfusion. And many were eager to do it. There may have been some psychological benefit in watching "bad blood" pouring out into a measuring bowl, but little physiological basis—except in certain cases of heart failure*—has ever been offered for this unusual practice that flourished so widely for hundreds of years. It undoubtedly killed many patients who might have recovered if left to themselves.

THE BREAKTHROUGH: WILLIAM HARVEY

Transfusion in the modern sense—direct injection into the circulatory system of the patient—did not begin until the seventeenth century. It was William Harvey, with his discovery and description of the circulation of the blood in 1616, first published in *De Motu Cordis* (1628), who laid the theoretical foundation and made possible all subsequent advances.[4] Harvey's work was one of the triumphs of early modern science and helped spur the scientific revolution that came to dominate European intellectual life during the second half of the seventeenth century.

Harvey was the first person to provide a clear picture of the circula-

---

*In certain types of congestive heart failure, when there is too much fluid in the lungs, bloodletting can be effective.

tion of the blood—the process by which nutrients, respiratory gases, and metabolic wastes are transported through the living organism. Previously, the heart and arteries were considered a separate system from the liver and veins. It was believed that the veins carried nutritive blood from the liver to all parts of the body. Harvey was trying to explain why the veins, which transmitted so much blood to the arteries in only one direction, did not become quickly drained, and why the arteries, which received all this blood, did not burst. He speculated that only if the blood somehow returned from the arteries to the veins at the periphery could this phenomenon be explained. And it was the metaphor of a circle—a lightning bolt of inspiration—that led him to his original conception of this circular, continuous movement of the blood: "I began to consider whether the blood might have a kind of motion, as it were, in a circle, and this I afterward found to be true."[5]

Harvey succeeded in showing that there was a single, closed system of organized vessels through which the blood moved and a single, all-important pump, the heart, that propelled the blood continuously through the vessels. Blood was carried away from the heart through the arteries (which replaced the veins as the principal blood-distributing vessels). These large arteries branched into progressively smaller channels until they reached the capillaries, a network of microscopic vessels.* It was at the site of the capillaries that the crucial exchange of oxygen and wastes took place. The capillaries then coalesced into veins and these vessels returned the blood to the heart.

This schema, apparently so simple and so familiar to us, was one of those rare breakthroughs in knowledge, a dazzling moment of illumination that has lit the path of modern physiology and science ever since.

THE EARLY PIONEERS

Harvey's discovery spurred great interest in transfusion. Around 1656, Sir Christopher Wren—who began as an astronomer and anatomist before settling on architecture—showed that dogs could be

---

*Harvey's discovery was all the more impressive because he lacked the tools— Leeuwonhoek's microscope did not appear until the 1670s—to actually see the capillaries. He merely deduced their presence and established them as the missing link between the veins and arteries.

given drugs and liquid intravenously more effectively than by mouth. Soon Wren, Sir Robert Boyle, and others were experimenting with intravenous infusions: beer, wine and opium were among the substances they attempted to introduce into the bloodstream.

The first successful transfusion, from the artery of one dog to the vein of another, was performed in 1665 by Richard Lower of Oxford.[6] The recipient dog had almost bled to death, but Lower's transfusion saved him. Encouraged by his success with canines, Lower decided to turn his efforts to humans.

Two years later, in October 1667, in front of the Royal Society of London—the occasion is recorded in Pepys' *Diary*[7]—Lower performed a successful transfusion of sheep's blood on one Arthur Conga, a 22-year-old member of the clergy "somewhat unbalanced, whose brain was considered a little too warm."[8] It was hoped the operation would alter his character.

Conga "was willing to suffer the experiment of transfusion to be tryed upon himself for a guiny."[9] Six to seven ounces were bled from his vein and then he was connected via silver tubes and quills to a sheep's carotid artery. In two minutes, nine to ten ounces of sheep's blood were transfused into his body. Afterward, the patient "found himself very well"[10] and six days later he gave the Society a talk in Latin describing how much better he felt. Given what we know today about transfusion reactions and incompatibility between animal and human blood, this was a truly astonishing event, a good example of a patient surviving despite his treatment.

In July of the same year, 1667—a few months before Lower's transfusion*—Jean-Baptiste Denis of France, philosopher and physician to Louis XIV, performed the first well-documented, successful human transfusion.[11] Denis transfused a 15-year-old boy who was suffering from febrile illness, and from anemia and exhaustion due to repeated bloodletting, with 9 ounces of sheep's blood and cured him of his ailment. Heartened by his success, Denis next used a healthy, paid volunteer who received 20 ounces of sheep's blood. Despite registering "very great heat" along the vein in his arm, the subject felt so strong afterward that he proceeded to butcher the sheep and go drinking with his companions.

---

*For years, the French and English, in their inimitable, competitive fashion, disputed who should get credit for performing the first transfusion. Although the international debate was never fully resolved, it is generally acknowledged today that Lower of England performed the first successful animal transfusions while Denis of France was first with human transfusions.

Denis's next subject did not fare so well. A lunatic subject to vio-
lent, maniacal fits, the man died after his third transfusion in two
months. The man's wife, spurred on by Parisian physicians, brought
formal charges against Denis, claiming that the transfusion had killed
her husband. (His fellow physicians were not only jealous of Denis
but feared criticism for their own practice of bleeding and purging.)

Although Denis was exonerated at the trial—the defense proved
that the man had been poisoned with arsenic by his wife!—the resulting furor led to the banning of transfusion experiments in France.
The English Parliament followed with its own prohibition a short
time later, and the magistrates in Rome soon joined them. For the
next 150 years, all public interest and experiment in transfusion
disappeared—a truly remarkable setback and an immeasurable loss
for science and medicine.

During this 150-year Dark Age for transfusion, there were two
important discoveries in related fields. In 1774, Joseph Priestley demonstrated the role of blood in carrying oxygen from the lungs to the
tissues, and in 1777 Antoine-Laurent Lavoisier clarified the nature of
oxygen and its role in respiration. Returning to Harvey's model of the
circulatory system, it is now possible to round out the picture of the
basic role of blood.

The heart is divided into four chambers. Circulated blood returns
from the veins through the two chambers on the right side, carrying
the waste product carbon dioxide. This blood is bluish because it has
lost its oxygen, which normally gives blood its red color. The returning blood passes through the right atrium or collecting chamber and
into the right ventricle, which pumps it into the lungs where carbon
dioxide is expelled while the blood is recharged with fresh oxygen.

This red, oxygen-rich blood is then collected into the left atrium. It
is held in this reservoir for less than a second before being pumped
into the left ventricle—the most powerful chamber in the heart; its
job is to pump blood to all parts of the body. The left ventricle,
working at 60 to 80 beats per minute, sends the freshly oxygenated
blood through the arteries to the capillaries, where it distributes
oxygen to the body and picks up carbon dioxide. As blood gives up
oxygen and picks up carbon dioxide, it turns from red to blue again.
The spent bluish blood then returns to the heart and the lungs, where
it loses its carbon dioxide and picks up oxygen, beginning the cycle
again. The average blood cell takes about one minute to return to its
starting point in this cycle.

These eighteenth century discoveries provided a fuller understanding of the blood and so, indirectly, helped pave the way for transfusion as a future mode of therapy.

THE NINETEENTH CENTURY: TRANSFUSION REVIVED

James Blundell, a pioneering English obstetrician, revived medical interest in transfusion in the nineteenth century. Blundell was frustrated by the number of his female patients who suffered serious and often fatal hemorrhages during childbirth. Around 1817 to 1818, he experimented on dogs and found that death from hemorrhage could be prevented by transfusion with blood from other dogs. Although it seems self-evident to us today, Blundell was the first person to make an explicit connection between blood loss and recovery through transfusion. It seems never to have occurred to anyone before that blood lost through injury or disease could be directly replaced with new blood via transfusion.

Blundell also found that blood taken from the vein was just as effective as arterial blood. He used a syringe and noted that it facilitated the operation, giving him more time and freedom for transfusion without harming the blood. Most importantly, it was James Blundell who first stated that species lines could not be crossed. For humans, "only human blood should be employed."[12]

Blundell transfused ten seriously ill patients with human blood and saved five of them. These were the first real transfusions since Denis and Lower, and the first transfusions ever between human and human. Blundell's new insights, his technique, and the special instruments he devised were far advanced for their day, but he had a falling out with Guy's Hospital in London and retired at 48 without the recognition he deserved.

Other physicians followed Blundell's lead, refining his technique and improving his apparatus: better needles, valves, and syringes were devised. But transfusion remained dangerous because there was no understanding of blood groups and incompatibility and no remedy for blood clotting. Severe and even fatal reactions were frequent. The risk of infection was also high until Joseph Lister introduced the use of antiseptics in 1867 and sterilization of instruments became mandatory.

Throughout the nineteenth century, transfusion was used only spo-
radically and often as a last resort. Despite Blundell's strictures—and
Leonard Landois's conclusive studies in 1878[13]—attempts to transfuse animal blood did not totally disappear. During the American
Civil War, two injured soldiers were reputed to have undergone successful transfusions of human blood;[14] they were lucky, for most transfusions were a hit-or-miss operation, killing at least as many patients
as they saved, since there was no knowledge of human blood types or
groups.

In an effort to find a less dangerous substance than blood for
transfusions, milk was briefly championed for intravenous therapy.
The idea was based on an old theory that milk could be converted
into white blood corpuscles. During a cholera epidemic in the 1860s
two out of five patients transfused with cow's milk survived. Later
goat's milk was also tried. T. G. Thomas, a strong advocate of milk
transfusions, predicted a "brilliant and useful future for intravenous
lacteal injections," claiming that "milk is more allied to chyle, the
material of which nature makes blood."[15] Some enthusiasts predicted
milk would supersede blood for transfusions. But after 1880, and
increasingly poor results, the advocacy of milk subsided. As with
animal blood, there is no telling how many deaths went unreported
until the absurdity of this practice was recognized.

Another substitute for blood that did catch on—and is still used
today—was intravenous isotonic saline (salt) solution. Saline was the
first reasonably safe replacement for moderate blood loss. It was
found to be simpler to inject and far safer to absorb than blood. In
cases of blood loss, saline works by thinning out the remaining blood
and allowing it to reach essential parts of the body. Vital organs like
the heart, brain, and kidneys need a constant supply of blood to
survive, and the human body will tolerate thinned-out blood sooner
than no blood at all. Thus salt solutions became an extremely popular
substitute, which led to the virtual abandonment of blood transfusion
at the end of the nineteenth century.

LANDSTEINER AND BLOOD GROUPS

At the start of the twentieth century—in the year 1900—Karl
Landsteiner of Vienna made the single most important discovery in
the history of blood transfusion. Landsteiner demonstrated that
there were different human blood groups and that consideration of

these differences was essential in choosing compatible blood for transfusion. This advance, for which Landsteiner won a Nobel Prize, remains the cornerstone of all transfusion therapy today. It has also given birth to the new science of immunohematology, while advancing the knowledge of genetics, anthropology, and forensic medicine, among other fields.

Landsteiner investigated the reactions between the red cells and serum of 22 individuals.[16] He found that the sera of certain people would clump or agglutinate the red blood cells of certain others. More specifically, the serum of one person may contain "isoagglutinins" that will react with corresponding "agglutinogens" on the red cells of some other person. Based on these differences, Landsteiner divided human blood into four major groups, which were designated A, B, AB, and O—an effective international nomenclature still in use today.*

Landsteiner's classification system works in this way: the serum of a group A person will agglutinate or clot the red cells of group B, because the A serum contains an anti-B isoagglutinin. Conversely, the isoagglutinin in the serum of a group B person will clot the red blood cells of persons in group A. Translated into practical language: groups A and B are incompatible and should never donate blood to one another. Transfusing type A blood to a type B person will cause massive clotting—in the form of microscopic clots disseminated throughout the body—and usually death.

A person with type A blood can donate to another person with type A blood, or to someone with type AB blood. A person with type B blood can donate to another individual with type B or to one with AB. A person with type AB can donate blood only to another type AB but, as the "universal recipient," can receive blood from all the other

---

*Landsteiner originally found three blood groups, which he called A, B, and C (now O). Two years later, two of his students, experimenting on a larger, more varied group, confirmed his first findings and also discovered the existence of a fourth, rare blood type, AB. Today, while these four major groups still obtain, more sophisticated techniques have identified 600 or more relevant subtypes—of which about 25 are known to be clinically significant—making true compatibility a delicate, difficult task. Another major subdivision is the Rh blood group, otherwise known as the Rh factor. The Rh factor was originally discovered in the blood of Rhesus monkeys. People who are Rh-positive (who have the Rh factor) can receive blood from either Rh-positive or Rh-negative persons, but Rh-negative people can receive blood only from other Rh-negative individuals. About 90 percent of the U.S. population is Rh-positive.

types: A, B, AB, and O. Finally, a type O individual, known as the "universal donor," can donate blood to all four types but can receive blood only from another person with type O.

Prior to Landsteiner and the classification of blood groups, a random transfusion between any two people carried a 35 percent likelihood of incompatibility. This led to agglutination and hemolysis or rupture of the red cells—a serious, potentially fatal result. The discovery of isoagglutination—of immunologic incompatibility—helped explain the mystery of transfusion reactions and fatalities encountered in early transfusion experiments. It was now understood for the first time that donor and recipient must be of similar, or compatible, blood types. Blood grouping and cross matching subsequently became essential preliminaries, and much of the danger of previous random transfusions was eliminated.

Although Landsteiner established a system to make transfusion safe and effective, many years passed before his findings were put to practical use. Reuben Ottenberg probably performed the first blood transfusions in New York City in 1907 and 1908. He initiated the typing and cross-matching of donors and recipients before transfusion and, despite some opposition, made it a standard hospital procedure. Ottenberg also introduced the concept of the "universal donor," showing that group O blood could be given to recipients of the other three types—a vital contribution for emergency transfusions.[17]

BLOOD CLOTTING AND ANTICOAGULATION

Following Landsteiner, the second crucial breakthrough in transfusion medicine—and the other major advance of the twentieth century—was the discovery of a safe, effective anticoagulant.

Unlike blood groups and incompatibility, the problem of blood clotting was long recognized as a major handicap to transfusion. It was well known that blood tended to clot within a few minutes of leaving the protection of the blood vessels. If it was not immediately infused, its flow was impeded and it became a useless coagulated mass. The only solution seemed to be direct transfusion: to connect the blood vessels of donor and recipient so that outside exposure was limited and blood flow remained smooth and continuous.

Initially, in animal-to-animal and animal-to-man transfusions, the donor's artery was connected to the recipient's vein. This method exploited the pump action of the heart to generate a forceful, rapid flow and thus avoid stagnation and clotting. However, when human donors became more common in the nineteenth century and vein-to-vein transfusions were used, clotting became an even more serious impediment to the transfer of adequate amounts of blood.

Various devices and ingenious strategies were adopted to circum- vent this problem. One popular remedy, used in American hospitals until the 1920s, was transfusion of defibrinated blood: blood in which some of the key clotting elements have been removed. Blood was collected in an open vessel and allowed to clot. Then it was whipped up—with a wire egg beater—until the clot was strained out and re- moved. The clot-free liquid blood was then injected into the patient. This was a poor method, for it ruptured the cells—by breaking up the connective fibrin—and injured the blood.

For a short period around the turn of century, direct transfusion via artery-to-vein anastomoses came into vogue.[18] Anastomosis in- volved the delicate surgical connection of veins and arteries into a continuous channel. Only the most skillful, and hence celebrated, surgeons could perform this complex suturing.

The French Nobel Prize winner Alexi Carrel was the champion of this method; in 1908, he won mass publicity when he used it to save a five-day-old girl in New York by anastomosing her to her father in an emergency operation performed on the kitchen table. Another anas- tomosis advocate was the Cleveland surgeon G. W. Crile, who devised a metal tube through which the recipient's vein could be pulled. The vein was rolled back and tied over the end of the tube so that the donor's artery could more easily be sewn with it. Crile performed 61 transfusions with this method and reported his results in 1909, in the first book on transfusion in America.[19]

These methods of direct transfusion all had the same drawback: the donor's physical presence was mandatory. They also required large teams of trained personnel. In anastomosis, another difficulty was determining how much blood had been transfused (one crude tech- nique was simply to weigh the donor before and after). Often, too, both recipient and donor developed complications. Less direct or "mediate" methods, using vein-to-vein transfusions with syringes, were tried next. These had the advantage of measuring the exact amount of blood transfused. But they too were dependent on "syringe specialists" and were hampered by the same direct person- to-person approach.

The discovery of a chemical to overcome blood clotting was thus an urgent priority. It had long been established through direct observation that ordinary table salt could temporarily keep blood from clotting. In 1890, two Swiss scientists, André Arthus and Germaine Pages, had related calcium to blood clotting and shown that small amounts of calcium salts would keep blood fluid so that it could be injected into animals. But the practical value of their findings was ignored for over 20 years, until a new wave of interest arose around the beginning of World War I.

In 1914, several scientists worldwide—in Belgium, Argentina, and America—simultaneously began experimenting with sodium citrate and glucose as an anticoagulant for blood. They demonstrated that blood could be withdrawn into a container and mixed with citrate to prevent clotting before it was transfused through a process called *chelation* (the chemical binding of calcium to blood which inhibits its clotting action). At first this worked for only a few minutes, but it was startling nonetheless.

In 1915, Richard Lewisohn showed that a minimum of 0.2% citrate would prevent blood clotting for several hours. Lewisohn perfected the technique and standardized the dosage of sodium citrate, thus paving the way for a far simpler and safer mode of transfusion.[20] This discovery of an effective anticoagulant led to the "indirect method" of blood transfusion and revolutionized the field, opening up new possibilities that are still being explored today.

Once blood could be collected, preserved, and administered at separate sites, donor and recipient no longer had to lie side by side in the operating room or on the kitchen table. Freed from this major limitation, blood transfusion therapy could develop into the widespread lifesaving practice that it is today—and into a major, multi-billion-dollar industry. But before that happened, there were still more obstacles to overcome and new refinements to be made.

WARS AND PROGRESS

It is one of the savage ironies in the twentieth century history of blood transfusion that many of the greatest advances occurred during wartime. While unprecedented volumes of blood were being spilled, scientists were simultaneously engaged in pioneering research to preserve this vital fluid and make it more widely and easily available.

One of the most important medical discoveries of World War I was that blood could resuscitate victims of hemorrhagic shock—a condition wherein the patient loses so much blood that the vital areas of the body are deprived of oxygen.* Since 70 to 80 percent of battle wounds are accompanied by shock, the adequate supply of transfusable blood to the front lines became an urgent matter. In 1917, O. H. Robertson, a Canadian medical officer, introduced the use of a citrate-glucose solution of the same volume as the blood being collected. The citrate prevented clotting by removing ionized calcium from the blood, while the glucose, in tandem with ice box refrigeration, permitted storage for 7 to 14 days.

Robertson's method was unwieldy, requiring the long-distance transport of huge volumes of fluid to the battlefields and base hospitals, but the blood plus the citrate-glucose solution saved many from posthemorrhagic shock. This was the first attempt at anticoagulation and refrigeration for short-term preservation of whole blood. In 1918, the prescient Robertson stated that blood could be stored for up to 21 days—but he was ignored until another war came along and forced medical science to advance despite itself.[21]

The Spanish Civil War (1936–39) was the next occasion for the development and refinement of blood transfusion. Blood was collected from civilians and stored under refrigeration by the transfusion service of the Spanish Republican Army. It was transferred to casualty stations and base hospitals where it proved effective for treatment of the wounded. Transfusion records were also kept and grouping and cross-matching accurately practiced and checked.

The first civilian blood bank in the United States was organized by B. Fantus, at Cook County Hospital in Chicago in 1937. At this early date, refrigerated blood could be effectively used only seven to ten days. As a result, there was a high wastage of unused blood, and blood banking was thus uneconomical except in large hospitals where daily transfusion demands justified all the work and preparation. There was as yet no well-organized voluntary U.S. blood service, as there was in Great Britain, where a network of regional centers and a "walking-donor service" had been established since 1921.

World War II created a critical need for blood and led to the rapid expansion of blood-collecting agencies. This huge wartime effort focused mainly on plasma: the fluid part of the blood that accounts for 55 percent of total blood volume. The immense value of plasma for

*Another advance was the selection of donors not only on the basis of blood group but good health and freedom from transmissible infectious diseases such as syphilis and malaria.

the treatment of shock was just being recognized at this time. Plasma can be stored for months either in a frozen state or as a dried powder since it does not deteriorate. When whole blood was not available, there were great advantages in using plasma.[22]

Great Britain began collecting plasma in 1939 and in June 1940 requested American aid for British and French casualties. A nation-wide program was initiated to enlist volunteer donors and ship the plasma abroad. In 1941, with America's entry into the war, the Red Cross began collecting plasma for the U.S. armed forces. By the end of the war, 13 million units had been collected in the first of the national "blood drives," an impressive achievement by any standard. Most of the plasma was shipped as a dried powder and then dissolved in sterile water for injection at the battlefront.

Another important development during World War II was the introduction of a new anticoagulant, acid-citrate-dextrose (ACD). E. L. Degowin with his associates in America and J. F. Loutit and P. L. Mollison in England developed a solution that could preserve blood for up to 21 days. By August 1944, the first whole blood shipments with ACD were sent to Europe and later they went to the Pacific as well. The new 21-day standard for preserving whole blood made transfusion easier, cheaper and more effective.

FRACTIONATION

Since the thirties, Edwin Cohn and his associates at Harvard had been experimenting with the fractionation or separation of plasma into useful derivatives.[23] When World War II began Cohn was still working on plasma derivatives drawn from animal blood. The U.S. Army, anticipating huge blood needs, pressed him for a safe and effective fluid replacement that could be transported to the battlefield.

Cohn discovered too many side effects from animal plasma so he switched to fractionating human blood. Early findings were encour-aging, but before he could complete his clinical studies, the Pearl Harbor attack occurred. In the ensuing crisis, human blood deriva-tives were flown in from Harvard and effectively used for American casualties. Within two years of these successful results, seven Ameri-can pharmaceutical companies were building commercial labora-tories to produce Cohn plasma fractions under Harvard's patent.

The ability to separate serum albumin was the first practical result of Cohn's fractionation process. Serum albumin, the most abundant protein in plasma, is the most essential ingredient in the treatment of shock since it helps to keep fluid in the bloodstream. Isolated from plasma, it offers several advantages: it is highly concentrated; it can be bottled in liquid form and shipped ready to use since it does not need to be reconstituted; and, perhaps most importantly, it can be purified of serum hepatitis, a serious threat that was becoming increasingly well documented and exists to this day.

Another product of Cohn's fractionation process was gamma globulin, a special group of proteins containing valuable antibodies against viruses and bacteria. When injected prophylactically, gamma globulin can protect against specific diseases for three to four weeks. Fibrinogen, which contains an important clotting factor, and Factor VIII, which can be vital to hemophiliacs, are two more useful derivatives of fractionated plasma.

Cohn's fractionation process is still in use today and it has clearly brought significant benefits to transfusion medicine. But the possibility of separating blood into "product" components has also led to certain excesses and abuses. A huge profit-making industry has sprung up to capitalize on the economic opportunities inherent in the marketing of plasma and other blood components, and it has sometimes acted against the best medical interests of the consumer. This "pharmaceutical sector" and its plasma operations—as well as its overlap with the Red Cross and other "whole blood" suppliers who later switched to component therapy—will be examined in the following two chapters.

POST-WAR: RAPID GROWTH OF A NEW INDUSTRY

After the war, the use of blood and blood products in transfusions expanded at a rapid pace. Physicians and surgeons who had come to rely on transfusions in wartime now called for civilian blood banks so that they could continue their successful use of transfusions in peacetime. The public had also become accustomed to making blood donations and was better prepared to participate in a national blood program. Hospital, community, and regional blood banks sprang up all across the country, with the Red Cross and the AABB taking a leading role. The whole blood services complex as we know it today was largely a result of the Second World War and the changes it set in motion.

The fifties and sixties saw major advances in techniques for the preservation of human blood. For many years, blood commonly had been withdrawn through rubber tubing and collected into glass bottles. This led to the rapid deterioration of red cells and presented a serious obstacle to long-term storage. Due to continued reuse, bottles and rubber stoppers also caused a high incidence of pyrogenic, or fever, reactions. In the early fifties, disposable plastic tubes and plastic collecting bags were developed. This advance ensured a safer, cleaner, and more flexible system for storing and preserving blood.

In 1957, a new preservative, citrate-phosphate-dextrose (CPD) was introduced by J. G. Gibson and his associates. CPD extended the storage period of blood from 21 to 28 days, with a loss of less than 30 percent of the red cells (the maximum allowed at the time by the Division of Biologic Standards of the NIH). CPD was also less acid and so reduced the storage lesions of the red cells in the collecting bags. Most blood banks converted to CPD as a preservative solution, though the dating period by government regulations was maintained at a conservative 21 days.

In 1940 Basile Luyet and Marie Pierre Gehenio published their classic treatise, *Life and Death at Low Temperatures,* and thereby gave birth to the new field of cryobiology. In 1951, Audrey Smith observed that glycerol protects red cells from the lethal effects of freezing and so opened new possibilities for long-term preservation of blood. In the 1960s, techniques for freezing red cells were developed that allowed long-term storage and stockpiling of blood for the first time.[24] Plasma was separated from red cells by a high-speed centrifuge, and then the red cells were brought to subfreezing temperatures with the aid of cryoprotective agents like glycerol. Storage with this method could last for as long as 10 to 20 years. Thawing and washing techniques permitted recovery for most (75 to 90 percent) of the frozen red cells. This unfrozen blood could then be successfully transfused—a truly remarkable innovation.

In addition to long-term storage and stockpiling of blood for emergencies or wars, freezing allowed for the preservation of rare blood types and large quantities of group O, "universal donor" blood. Frozen red cells also guaranteed the absence of reaction-causing leukocytes* and plasma and a far lower risk of hepatitis infection.

These important advantages were offset by higher costs. The process of freezing blood required more time for preparation, more storage space, more expendable supplies, and a larger staff. Yet,

---

*Leukocytes are the white blood cells that fight infection.

despite these drawbacks, frozen blood has been used increasingly and has proved itself in the one area that counts: improving patient care. Today it still holds the greatest hope for purity, safety, and effectiveness—and the only hope for indefinite storage.

The improvements in preservation technology made large quantities of blood available for the first time, and this in turn led to great advances in open-heart surgery, organ transplantation, and other complicated operations, previously considered too long or too dangerous. Open heart surgery requires two to eight pints of blood—and occasionally more—and would have been unthinkable without an ample ready supply of blood. Other types of delicate surgery on the brain, lungs, and blood vessels also became feasible.

But these innovative procedures using vast quantities of blood also created new problems. One that still plagues the transfusion process today is the use of multiple donors. Since a healthy person may only donate one unit of blood every eight weeks, and since refrigerated blood becomes outdated after a maximum of 42 days, it takes many different donors to make up a fresh multiunit supply of blood. Each of these multiple donors must be cross-matched against all the other donors, as well as against the recipient, to avoid an immunologic reaction. There is a high degree of variability between the blood constituents of any two individuals and a 1 in 50 chance of some kind of reaction, usually relatively mild but occasionally severe and even life-threatening. With 600 known types and subtypes of blood—as opposed to Landsteiner's 4—the chances of an untoward reaction increase geometrically when a large pool of donors is involved.

TRANSFUSION TODAY: COMPONENT THERAPY

In the late sixties, it became increasingly common to separate whole blood into its constituent parts and use each component separately. Red cells, white cells, platelets, and plasma were injected specifically and independently of one another. This method of component therapy was found to be more economical in conserving the supply of blood and for certain conditions, such as chronic anemia, it was also more effective: the anemic patient needs only red cells and has no use for plasma, which can overload his circulation.

In other cases, however, the use of component therapy is more questionable. When a person bleeds, he or she loses whole blood with all its components. To replace only one of these specific components, such as the red cells, while leaving out the plasma and platelets, which have also been lost, cannot be in the patient's best interest. But it is far more economical, since one unit of whole blood can produce two or more components that sell for a higher price than the original unit.

Today component therapy has become so widespread that whole blood is rarely used: from 1971 to 1980 whole-blood transfusion declined from 67 percent of the total to only 13 percent. Today it is less than 6 percent.[25] While blood is now capable of producing numerous useful by-products—the latest count is 17 preparations from a single unit—the profit motive has perhaps played too determining a role in this near-exclusive reliance on blood components rather than whole blood.

Though progress was slow and halting for the first 300 years after Harvey's discovery of the principle of circulation, since World War II blood transfusion therapy has grown and expanded impressively. Important improvements have been registered in blood typing and matching, preservation, fractionation, and the increasingly sophisticated and specific treatment of illness and injury. Major advances in surgery and treatment would have been impossible without these developments. Human blood, that mysterious "spirit" of the ancients, the chief "humor" of the medievals, has come to play a much larger, more diverse, and more indispensable role in saving life than anyone ever dreamed. At the same time, the widespread reliance on transfusions has made the safety of the blood supply a vital issue for millions of Americans. We can no longer take that safety for granted.

3

The Blood Supply I:
The Voluntary Sector
and Nonprofit
Organizations

Think of us as tax-exempt rather than not-for-profit. We have to make a profit.

Gilbert Clark, Director of the American Association of Blood Banks

Three organizations in the United States collect whole blood for the entire country. Of these three, the American Red Cross (ARC) is by far the largest, the wealthiest, and the most powerful. The Red Cross, America's official voluntary relief agency, entered the civilian blood market at the end of World War II. Today it operates 56 regional centers across the United States, supplying one-half of the nation's donated blood to hospitals.[1] The undisputed leader in the blood services field, the American Red Cross has also enjoyed an historically close and significant relationship with the federal government.

The Red Cross's rival and longtime competitor is the American Association of Blood Banks (AABB), a trade group of over 2,000 hospitals and community blood centers. The AABB was formed in 1947 to protect the interests of independent hospital blood banks against the monopolistic intentions of the Red Cross. Today about 25 percent of the country's blood is collected through the AABB.[2]

A third organization, the Council of Community Blood Centers (CCBC) is a smaller trade group of mostly regional blood banks. Originally a breakaway group within the AABB, today the CCBC accounts for 20 percent of blood collections and is more closely allied with the Red Cross than with the AABB.[3] A relative newcomer to the blood services complex—it was established in 1962—the CCBC has played a minor role compared to the Red Cross and the American Association of Blood Banks.

These three organizations have overlapping memberships. Thus all but two of the CCBCs 31 regional centers are also part of the AABB, which is a loose confederation, compared to the tighter corporate structure of the Red Cross.

The Red Cross, the AABB, and the CCBC are referred to as the "voluntary sector" because they take donations from unpaid volunteers.* They are officially classified as "not-for-profit" organizations and as such have a tax-exempt status. But as already discussed in Chapter 1, this designation has not prevented them from becoming highly profitable, particularly in the case of the Red Cross. In 1986, in an article which won the National Magazine Award for Journalism in the Public Interest, reporter Andrea Rock revealed the substantial profits that tax exempt corporations earn from the blood business:[5]

> If the Red Cross Blood Services were a for-profit corporation, its fiscal 1985 revenues would place it in the Fortune 500 position at No. 473. Its 8.8% excess of revenues over expenses for that year would put it in a tie with Philip Morris for 50th place among Fortune 500 firms in terms of net income as a percentage of sales. Other blood banking organizations are generally profitable, though on a smaller scale.[6]

Rock pointed out that the huge "excess funds" from the Red Cross Blood Services did not go toward research or other charitable Red Cross activities. Often they don't even finance the Blood Services' own expansion. In one example cited by Rock, the Red Cross was trying to raise donations from the public to pay for a planned $17

*In 1970, over 10 percent of whole blood units were from paid donors. By 1980, this figure was down to 2.2 percent.[4] However, the voluntary sector also depends on commercial pharmaceutical firms to manufacture derivatives from its recovered and salvaged plasma. The business of collecting and fractionating plasma—the tax-paying plasma industry, which relies heavily on paid donors—functions as a separate enterprise and will be considered in the next chapter.

million research facility in Rockville, Maryland. Instead of support-
ing such projects, the Red Cross surplus revenue "goes to a balance-
sheet category called accumulated net assets." These net assets make
the Red Cross Blood Services "a very rich organization."[7]

Clearly, nonprofit blood collecting is a lucrative enterprise
wherein economic self-interest plays a larger role than might be expected. Hard-headed, bottom-line economics has long influenced the
policies of the blood industry and it continues to do so today—even
though it is often couched in misleading moralistic terms. A review of
the history and development of the voluntary sector—and of the Red
Cross's leading role within it—enables us to understand better why
the quality of our blood supply is not as high today as it should be.

"THE GREATEST MOTHER IN THE WORLD"

The first multilateral agreement creating the International Red Cross
was signed at the Geneva Conference in 1864, which was attended by
delegates from 16 countries.

The agreement committed member governments to care for all
casualties during war, be they allies or enemies. The driving force
behind this new humanitarian concept was Jean-Henri Dunant, a
Swiss banker who organized emergency aid services for Austrian and
French wounded at the Battle of Solferino in 1859.* In 1862, Dunant
wrote about the needless sufferings he had witnessed in a much-
publicized book, *Un Souvenir de Solferino,* where he proposed the formation of voluntary relief societies in all countries. Dunant's novel
idea was to have specially organized relief committees visit the battlefield, flying their own flag to identify themselves as politically neutral
while they dispensed aid to the victims of both sides. With the Geneva
Convention of 1864, Dunant's flag—a red cross on a white field—was
adopted as an international standard.

The American Red Cross was established in 1881 by Clara Barton,
famed as "the angel of the battlefields" for her relief work with
wounded soldiers during both the American Civil War and the
Franco-Prussian War of 1870. In 1882, after several attempts, she
succeeded in having the United States sign the Geneva Agreement.

---

*During the Crimean War in 1854, Florence Nightingale had first demonstrated that
the wounded should not be left behind for dead but could survive with basic sanitary
assistance.

Later she authored the American amendment to the constitution of the Red Cross: this amendment enlarged the Red Cross's mandate to dispense aid not only in war but for disaster relief as well.

For many years, Barton campaigned tirelessly to win a federal charter for her group—based in Washington, D.C.—while she fought off competition by rival Red Cross societies in other states. In 1900, her efforts were rewarded when the American National Red Cross was officially incorporated by an act of Congress. The charter of 1900 legitimated Barton's group by giving it the exclusive right to provide volunteer aid to the wounded during war and to furnish relief aid for disaster victims. It established the American Red Cross as a national institution with formal government sanction, although never with any direct federal funding.

Barton herself served as the first president of the American Red Cross until 1904, when she retired as a result of a feud with a rival faction led by Mabel Boardman. Boardman became the new president of the American Red Cross following the personal intervention of President Theodore Roosevelt, thus establishing a tradition of close presidential involvement with the organization.[8] In 1905, a second act of incorporation formalized the role of the president in Red Cross affairs. Under this statute, amended in 1947, the president was to appoint eight of the Red Cross's fifty-member board of governors, including the principal officer of the corporation. The president himself was to act as the honorary chairman.

In 1905, Roosevelt selected William Howard Taft as principal officer of the Red Cross. Taft occupied a room adjoining the White House in this capacity. Later, Taft would move into the White House himself. Under Woodrow Wilson's administration, the new American Red Cross headquarters was built on government property facing the White House South Lawn. After World War II, Harry Truman appointed George Marshall to this important post, and later Richard Nixon chose Frank Stanton. The close relationship between the White House and the Red Cross persists to this day. In the 1986–87 annual report of the American Red Cross, President Reagan was listed as the honorary chairman, Ed Meese the honorary counselor, and Don Regan honorary treasurer. The secretaries of State, Defense, and Education, and the chairman of the Joint Chiefs of Staff were among the ruling governors.[9]

Under the provisions of its charter, the Red Cross was also required to submit an annual report of its finances to Congress for auditing. The government was thus able to ensure public accountability and a stricter degree of control over Red Cross activities. Because of these various ties to Washington, the Red Cross has often been referred to as a quasi-official arm of the government.

From 1900 on, the newly empowered Red Cross would zealously protect its exclusive privileges in an effort to maintain and expand its original mandate. In 1911, the Red Cross gained a significant victory when William Howard Taft designated it as the "only" society authorized to dispense aid during war. A little later, the U.S. Army agreed to assist Red Cross personnel and transport its supplies free of charge. Over the years, the Red Cross was to show great ingenuity and political skill in using its relationship with the government to win favorable regulations and policies.

IN SEARCH OF NEW MISSIONS

The Red Cross assumed its national character under Mabel Boardman, with a nationwide network of local chapters led by volunteers. This voluntary structure created problems for the Red Cross, which was expected by the public to function smoothly and efficiently like any official organization. However, the Red Cross had no duties to discharge in the long intervals between wars and disasters.[10] It was hard for the organization to keep itself going and attract volunteers during these lulls, and even harder to mobilize suddenly and efficiently during emergencies without an ongoing, operational structure.

Clearly the Red Cross needed a new defining mission beyond emergency relief to justify its existence on an everyday basis. In search of an expanded role, the Red Cross ventured into rural public health as early as 1907. Later it undertook to teach water safety, to care for the elderly, and to visit the sick.

These forays into new activities, however, led to clashes with other voluntary organizations that had already staked out the various areas as their territory. Before World War I the Red Cross sold TB stamps but later had to cede this role to the TB Society (now the American Lung Association). After World War I, the Red Cross came into direct conflict with the American Legion and the Veterans of Foreign Wars when it tried to provide aid to wounded veterans. When it sought to teach first aid and swimming, the Red Cross antagonized the YMCA and YWCA. The Salvation Army, the Volunteers for America, the

USO, and the Army and Navy all clashed at one time or another with what they perceived as Red Cross encroachment into their domains.[11]

Within the Red Cross itself, there were debates and disagreements about which direction to pursue. In 1922, a major showdown pitted the strict constructionists, who wanted continued commitment to war and disaster relief, against the expansionists, who favored a broader mandate. The strict constructionists lost and the decision was taken to expand and diversify, provoking new tensions with existing public health groups.*

During the New Deal and into the thirties, the Red Cross came up against its stiffest competitor and most formidable rival: the U.S. government. The new welfare state had far greater means and resources than any private charitable organization, and the Red Cross quickly lost ground in the face of the government's widespread public programs.

With the advent of World War II, the Red Cross found a new opportunity for expansion. In 1929 a transfusion service had first been proposed by local chapters but rejected by the national organization as not being "a proper Red Cross chapter activity."[13] Then, during the thirties, came the discovery that plasma could be effectively used to treat battlefield shock. As already noted, plasma could be shipped as a dried powder and reconstituted at the battlefield. In 1941, facing war, the U.S. armed services asked the American Red Cross to collect blood for the preparation of plasma. It was an urgent task and the Red Cross rose to it fully and impressively. By 1945, the American Red Cross collected 13 million pints of blood for U.S. forces and their allies through 35 regional and 63 mobile donor centers.[14]

The wartime blood program offered the Red Cross an extraordinary opportunity to extend its mandate to a permanent peacetime activity: a new civilian blood program. The Red Cross was uniquely qualified to run such a program; and there was sure to be a growing demand for blood following major therapeutic advances during the war. It appeared that the Red Cross had come upon the perfect solution to its perennial dilemma. A civilian blood service would not only sustain the Red Cross tradition of humanitarian aid, it would

*Competition also came from new Community Chest organizations who were "busy in an organized way biting 'the Greatest Mother' in the leg." President Roosevelt was called in to mediate this conflict and he backed the Red Cross, which was led by his friend and personal physician, Admiral Grayson.[12]

provide a big boost to the organization's public image by "keeping the Red Cross continuously in the minds of those upon whom it depends for support."[15]

Proceeding cautiously, the Red Cross consulted with all the relevant national authorities—the American Medical Association, the American Hospital Association, the U.S. Public Health Service, even the unions—before approving the concept of new civilian blood programs.* It continued to canvass endorsements through 1946 and 1947 from its local chapters. A Gallup poll in 1947 showed that 73 percent of those surveyed approved a national blood program under Red Cross management while 67 percent said they would donate. In June 1947, the new Red Cross blood service was formally approved by the Board of Governors. It was launched, amid great fanfare, in 1948.

THE RISE OF THE AABB

Almost immediately, the new Red Cross blood program encountered opposition and aroused controversy. For one, the Red Cross had vastly overestimated the civilian need for blood and fell far short of its targets.† Another problem arose from the local chapters that did not support the program or raise enough money. But the biggest setback came from individual communities, who strongly objected to the Red Cross takeover of local blood collection. Unlike the wartime program, which had been directly solicited by the government, the Red Cross made its own decision—and exceeded its statutory authority—in entering the civilian market.

In its preparatory consultation with national organizations, the Red Cross had neglected to consider community hospitals and civic groups who were already recruiting donors and drawing blood for local use. These rival blood banking groups, many established during the war, had no intention of disbanding for the benefit of the Red Cross. They resented the intrusion into their turf and they also felt

---

*The Red Cross actually approved *two* programs: a "national blood program" based on large regional centers and a second "permissive blood program" for individual Red Cross chapters on a community level. The two have coexisted uneasily, with frequent feuds and ruptures still plaguing the Red Cross today.[16]

†"The [Red Cross medical] advisers, implying careful calculation, had originally stated that domestic blood demand would quickly grow to five units per year per general medical and surgical bed. Later they admitted that there were no solid data upon which to base such a figure."[17]

threatened by basic ethical or "ideological" differences with the Red
Cross: not only was the Red Cross led by nonphysicians but it was
opposed to charging patients for blood they did not replace—a "nonreplacement fee," which these local hospitals and blood banks had
always charged.

Community blood groups decided to strike back, expanding and
opening up new centers themselves in order to preempt the Red
Cross. Since they did not have to coordinate their activities with a
national organization, they were able to act quickly, establishing
themselves solidly in the Southwest and Midwest before the Red
Cross program was officially launched. In November of 1947, leading
representatives from these groups met in Dallas and agreed to form
the American Association of Blood Banks as a direct response to the
Red Cross challenge.[18] Independent blood banks would henceforth
have an official organization to argue their case and defend their
interests on a national level.

Not only did the AABB become the chief rival of the Red Cross, it
also quickly established itself as the preeminent scientific leader in
blood banking. Many of its representatives, unlike those of the Red
Cross, were hematologists, pathologists, and other medical experts
from affiliated hospitals. These medical professionals gave the organization a clear scientific and technological edge. It was the AABB
which set the accepted standards for blood banking facilities, maintained files on rare blood types, and trained blood technicians at the
highest level.

Because it prided itself on being a scientific organization as well as
a trade group, the AABB was open to individual members along with
blood banking organizations. Even the Red Cross could join, although it repeatedly refused. Today, about 7,000 individual members, mostly blood banking personnel, belong to the AABB along
with over 2,300 institutions.[19]

Despite the membership of a small number of commercial banks,
the AABB is regarded primarily as a nonprofit entity. But, unlike the
Red Cross, it has long used the nonreplacement fee as an integral part
of its system. Under this requirement, a patient must "replace" the
amount of blood he receives from the hospital. He may donate it
himself or recruit a friend or relative to donate for him. If a patient
does not replace the blood he has received, he is charged for it,
usually at a rate between $25 and $50 a unit. In practice, many
patients would rather pay the fee than replace the blood; the result is

an important source of income for the AABB. On the other hand, the nonreplacement fee also acts as an incentive to donate.

In 1953 the AABB established a National Clearinghouse system to keep track of nonreplacement fees and other blood transactions. The clearinghouses, set up in a few major regions, facilitated the smooth flow of blood credits all across the country. A donor could build up predeposit credits that could offset any future fees he might incur. Alternatively, the donor could assign his credits to a friend or relative in another part of the country. In an emergency, this was a quick, efficient way of getting blood to someone in need. It also served to reward donors for their altruism.

The clearinghouse system helped make the AABB a national organization and a force to be reckoned with in the blood banking industry. In 1961, the Red Cross itself joined the Blood Clearinghouse Program, enhancing the program's resources and making it a truly nationwide system. It was also an indirect way of acknowledging the growing importance of the AABB.

INDIVIDUAL VERSUS COMMUNITY RESPONSIBILITY

Nevertheless, the Red Cross remained opposed to the AABB's use of a nonreplacement fee and blood credits. The Red Cross has long endorsed the position that blood should be given to any patient in need, regardless of his donating history. It rejects the idea of rewards of any kind and believes the giving of blood should be a community responsibility. Under this ideology, blood is thought of as common property: hence society is responsible for ensuring its availability to all, regardless of their participation.[20]

This position is neither as disinterested nor as charitable as it sounds, since the Red Cross itself always get paid. The onus of responsibility—and the burden of cost—still falls on the community. The economist Ross Eckert observes: "It is worth noting . . . that from the standpoint of the blood banks, a policy of volunteers-only amounts to setting a uniform maximum price—zero—on a key factor of production: this eliminates price competition in a manner analogous to setting a minimum price on the output of rival suppliers."[21] By eliminating the nonreplacement fee, the Red Cross was using a similar tactic against its chief competitor.

The AABB, on the other hand, supports a concept of individual

responsibility and has consistently opposed Red Cross efforts to so-
cialize blood resources and increase government regulation. According to the AABB, individuals should arrange to provide for their own
actual and potential blood needs—but should also receive preferen-
tial treatment for their contributions. This system offers effective
price breaks to those who replace blood and help maintain inventories. But it never gives money in any direct way. Rather, the *avoidance*
of a future nonreplacement fee becomes an incentive to donate
blood. The AABB assumes that individuals are more concerned with
protecting themselves and their families than with giving blood to the
community at large. (In practice, despite these ideological differences, people in immediate need always receive blood regardless of
their coverage or financial situation.)

The issue of the nonreplacement fee led to a split within the AABB
in 1962. Several of its larger blood banks opposed the fee but, because
of the one-member/one-vote rule, they were defeated by the smaller
but more numerous hospitals who did want it. Dissatisfied with the
dominance of the AABB by hospitals, six of the largest regional banks
split off and formed the Council of Community Blood Centers
(CCBC).[22] Though initially opposed to the Red Cross—and retaining
their membership in the AABB—the CCBC gradually became a Red
Cross ally. Today both advocate greater centralization and dominance of each region by a single collection agency. The CCBC also
supports the Red Cross in calling for community, as opposed to
individual, responsibility for the blood supply.[23]

The Red Cross and the AABB continued to clash and compete
during the 1960s. The Red Cross wanted higher fees in the Clearinghouse Program and it opposed AABB efforts to participate in Red
Cross emergency blood collections for the military. The AABB resented the continuing monopolistic efforts of the Red Cross and
chafed at the Red Cross failure to meet the blood needs in many of its
own regions. The two organizations also clashed over Medicare coverage.

THE GIFT RELATIONSHIP

In 1971 a British professor of social administration named Richard
Titmuss published a study of comparative blood systems called *The
Gift Relationship.*[24] Titmuss attacked the American practice of using
money and "blood insurance" as an incentive for donors, claiming

that this discouraged altruistic donors and attracted only those whose motive was financial gain. Paid donors often lied about their health and thereby caused an alarmingly high incidence of hepatitis in the American blood supply. The profit-minded approach, Titmuss said, also led to blood shortages.

According to Titmuss, the British blood supply was of much higher quality than the American precisely because there was no such payment system. As a result, more people were inclined to donate out of a sense of the larger social welfare. Titmuss criticized the materialistic culture of America where such a social conscience was lacking. He believed that blood had no place in the "economic market," where it was exchanged as a commodity by strangers; rather, it belonged in the "social market" as a gift or a moral transaction between members of society. His book, which the *New York Times* voted one of the seven best books of 1971, created new public awareness and concern about the quality of the blood supply and led to a major government review.

Titmuss's contention that cash blood was the ultimate cause of the high American rates of posttransfusion hepatitis was accepted without much protest at the time. Subsequent studies at the Mayo clinic, Massachusetts General Hospital, and the National Heart and Lung Institute have shown that commercial or cash blood is not intrinsically inferior to unpaid blood and can, in fact, be of higher quality.[25] At the Mayo clinic, select donors were paid to give blood regularly over a period of years. They registered the lowest rates of infection in the country, far lower than the nearest regional Red Cross center with its voluntary donors.

But Titmuss's original, somewhat moralistic indictment—he has been characterized as an authoritarian Fabian with an ideal social order in mind[26]—has stuck despite all evidence to the contrary. This devaluation of cash blood has become a useful shibboleth serving the leading nonprofit organizations.

In the 1970s, the Red Cross and the AABB both objected to market competition between cash and noncash blood, even though according to Titmuss noncash blood should have easily outperformed its rival. Knowing the public's concern with safety, the commercial firms would have made high quality blood from screened and registered donors a top priority and chief selling point. Competition is, after all, a basic premise of the free market system, which allows the consumer to demand the highest standards.

Yet such competition was never allowed. Demonstrating that cash and noncash blood were equally safe would have eroded the influence of nonprofit collectors.[27] Another danger was that cash payment might lure volunteer donors—and would-be volunteers—away from the Red Cross and the AABB to commercial blood banks, further undermining these nonprofit organizations.

Competition from cash blood also threatened one of the blood industry's most significant, and controversial, protections: its freedom from implied warranty and strict liability for any transfusion-related diseases, such as hepatitis or AIDS.

Under present statutes, providing blood is classified as a service rather than as the sale of a product. Therefore blood banks cannot be held liable for any injury or illness resulting from blood unless negligence can be proven. As Reuben Kessel, Titmuss's chief American critic and a major critic of the blood banking industry, has argued, this exemption has the startling effect of shifting responsibility from the blood bank to the patient.[28] It also reduces the incentive for blood banks to screen donors and blood more rigorously.

The blood industry gained its exemption from strict liability during the 1960s, before there was any test to screen for hepatitis. It argued that blood bankers should not be held liable for transmitting a disease they had no way of detecting. Now, however, with the new hepatitis tests available, this exemption seems unwarranted. It has also been applied to transfusion AIDS because of pressure from blood banks and the false impression that without such an exemption there would be serious blood shortages.[29] Meanwhile the blood industry has lobbied hard to persuade the courts that it must remain free from liability in order to fulfill its role of maintaining an adequate supply of blood.

The exemption from liability has allowed the industry to sidestep the principle of informed consent. Patients are not required to sign a document which warns that the average transfusion recipient has a 5 to 10 percent chance of contracting hepatitis and a .1 to .01 percent chance of contracting AIDS from his or her blood transfusions. Unlike the executives of any other company, blood bankers are not constrained from making claims—for example that the blood supply is virtually free from contamination—that could be used against them in a court of law. Since they are providing a service rather than a product, they are also absolved from any implied product warranty.

However, if there were open competition between cash and non-cash blood, nonprofit companies would have to provide guarantees of safety just as any commercial firm does. They could no longer skirt the issue of product liability or implied warranty. Instead, they would have to take the necessary measures to ensure that their blood was as safe as it could possibly be. Such measures would include a more selective donor pool possibly paid to encourage repeat donations, and the use of the patient's frozen blood. Malpractice insurance would also be necessary.

Under strict liability, the Red Cross, the AABB, and the CCBC could be held responsible for diseases and other adverse effects resulting from the blood they supplied. Such a change would require, at the least, a fundamental reorganization. According to Reuben Kessel:

> Imposing strict liability upon the volunteer agencies would be on a par with permitting the practice of nudism only in the polar regions; it is doubtful the cult could survive the rigors of this constraint. Since the supply of blood is the principal product line of the American Red Cross and many other groups . . . their place in the sun would either be eliminated or sharply reduced. Therefore it is not difficult to understand why both the hospitals and blood suppliers (and many hospitals are blood suppliers) oppose strict liability.[30]

The industry's opposition to any suggestion of liability is organized and effective. Throughout his Congressional term of service, from 1970 to 1976, Representative Ed Koch, later mayor of New York, was consistently opposed by the Red Cross and the AABB in his attempts to pass a bill that would have allowed taxpayers to claim the blood they had donated as a charitable contribution. The bill's sponsors conceived this as a way of encouraging the middle class to give blood and reduce shortages. However, the AABB was concerned that deductions and credits "would place a dollar value on blood itself."[31] (According to the IRS, gifts of money or property to charities are deductible, but services, including volunteer time and activities, are not.) The AABB wanted to preserve the principle that the giving of blood is a service. If blood were classified as a product, then blood banks would be exposed to strict liability for transfusion-transmitted disease. That was a risk that neither the AABB nor the Red Cross could afford to take. Koch never passed his bill.

With the advent of the AIDS crisis, however, blood banks have been challenged in a new way. The public has grown more informed, and less tolerant, of the blanket immunity long enjoyed by the blood industry. Today there are hundreds of pending lawsuits which allege that blood banks were negligent in keeping the AIDS virus out of the blood supply before 1985. The Red Cross has reportedly made several large out-of-court settlements on the provision that the documents remain sealed from public view and that the terms remain secret.[32] Even so, the courts have rarely ruled against the blood industry—or when they do, their decisions are quickly overturned.[33] Only recently have blood banks been held to a more stringent public account, though still only for negligence, not for product liability. The burden of proof is still on the patient, who must show that the blood bank neglected to provide adequate protection. The larger issue involves setting a legal precedent establishing that blood is a product that might harm the consumer and that blood banks should be responsible for its safety. While blood can never be a totally safe product— with the exception of one's own blood—the concern that multiple lawsuits might bankrupt blood banks should be balanced by the obligation of the blood bank to provide appropriate testing and screening procedures.

THE NATIONAL BLOOD POLICY

Titmuss's book, *The Gift Relationship,* which alerted the public to the dangers in the blood supply in 1971, also attracted the attention of Eliot Richardson, then secretary of Health, Education and Welfare. HEW was already aware of alarming reports that the blood supply might be as much as 15 to 20 percent contaminated. Richardson accepted Titmuss's basic thesis that paid blood accounted for the unacceptably low quality of the American blood supply and in 1973, in response to these growing concerns, HEW announced the National Blood Policy.

The aim of the National Blood Policy was to create "an all-voluntary blood donation system and to eliminate commercialism* in the acquisition of whole blood and blood components for transfusion therapy."[34] The idea was to improve the quality of the blood supply by relying on altruism, as Titmuss suggested; also to solicit volunteer blood only, banish paid blood, and reduce competition for donors through regionalization.

In 1975, the federal government established the American Blood

---

*The stricture against commercialism did not apply to plasma, which is still bought in the U.S. See next chapter.

Commission (ABC), an organization charged with implementing the National Blood Policy. It did not, however, invest this agency with any federal enforcement powers. The American Blood Commission was composed of the three major blood-collection groups, as well as health care providers like the American Medical Association and the Food and Drug Administration, and consumer groups like the American Legion, the AFL-CIO, and representatives from the commercial plasma industry. The ABC tried to act as a peacemaker and to reduce tensions among its rival factions. Since neither the Red Cross nor the AABB had managed to establish a single nationwide blood-banking system, it proposed to reduce competition for donors through regionalization. Each major area would have one recognized center responsible for all blood collection. By 1984, the ABC had approved 46 such regional associations across the nation accounting for 50 percent of collected blood.

The ABC also espoused a policy of resource-sharing by all parties in the blood services complex. It tried to link the AABB clearinghouse and the Red Cross, but the commercial sector objected because the Red Cross would not share its blood with them. The Red Cross quickly withdrew in fear that a suit would be filed and its substantial assets attacked in an antitrust action.[35]

Although it acts as a kind of coordinator for the blood industry and maintains an open dialogue among its members, the American Blood Commission has been hampered by internal disagreements—specifically between the Red Cross and the AABB on any major issue—and its own lack of enforcement power. Neither the voluntary nor commercial sectors are inclined to cede their independent powers to the ABC, and in 1983, the American Cancer Society and several other large agencies pulled out. Government funding also dried up and the commission has been forced to seek private support, with only limited success.

During the 1970s, the Red Cross and the AABB continued their ongoing rivalry. In 1972, the Red Cross formally voted to eliminate all replacement fees and move toward community responsibility. In 1976, it ended a term of 16 years in the AABB Clearinghouse, arguing, "It is wrong to buy and sell blood like cabbages."[36] The Red Cross withdrawal weakened the clearinghouse system—and its intended target, the AABB—but it also hurt the Red Cross in terms of public good will. Patients who had accumulated credits under the system were now denied their fair reward.

In 1977, under pressure from the Red Cross, the American Blood

Commission agreed that the U.S. blood supply should be maintained as a community responsibility without the use of a nonreplacement fee. This policy decision led to the estrangement of the AABB from the ABC. The Red Cross argued that American donors did not need a cash incentive, which only "cheapened" the act of giving blood to those who needed it.

By 1979, the AABB was formally complaining to Congress that the Red Cross was trying to eliminate the credit system—and by extension, the AABB—and "move blood banking toward a single, monolithic system."[37]

EXPANSION AND DIVERSIFICATION OF THE RED CROSS

In 1978, the American Red Cross appointed an ad hoc committee to evaluate its blood program and make policy recommendations. It was clear that some basic reassessment and a new direction was called for. After over 30 years in the business, the Red Cross understood that blood banking does not fit well in a voluntary organization. For one, it is a 24-hour, round-the-clock medical service, not an occasional event. Another problem is that blood banking is not a mandated Red Cross activity, like war and disaster relief. As a result, local chapters don't have to help with blood collection. Of 3,100 Red Cross chapters across the country, 1,800 voluntarily participate in the blood program. Such a dependence on chapter support causes great regional variability and tensions in management. There are additional strains between lay and medical staff and even some jealousy within the Red Cross because blood bankers earn the highest salaries.

In 1978 the Red Cross Blood Services recommended expanding and striking out in a wholly new direction. It agreed to meet 100 percent of the blood needs of the regions it served and, more dramatically, it decided to enter the market for blood plasma products, until then considered the sole province of commercial fractionators. But by this time it was evident that the demand for plasma and its derivatives was the fastest-growing and most lucrative part of the blood industry. Sales were already over a billion dollars annually and accelerating. The Red Cross proposal of a joint venture with the pharmaceutical giant Baxter-Travenol—an aggressively for-profit company—was an utterly unprecedented move. It showed the Red Cross's willingness to leave behind both the voluntary sector and its official ideology in a search for a larger share of the market. The Red Cross had decided to go into business in a big way.[38]

Today the Red Cross enjoys a contractual arrangement with a Baxter-Travenol subsidiary, Hyland Therapeutics. Hyland manufactures Red Cross donor plasma into derivatives that carry the Red Cross label. The Red Cross then sells its product in direct competition with commercial manufacturers like Revlon and Bayer. Red Cross Blood Services currently earns 15 to 20 percent of its annual revenues—around $80 million—through the sale of such plasma derivatives.

The Red Cross enjoys several advantages over its rival commercial firms. It was already noted that as a nonprofit organization, the Red Cross is exempt from paying taxes. Further, in keeping with its official ideology, it does not pay any fee to those who donate blood. For the commercial firms, these donor fees alone account for 30 percent of production costs. The Red Cross also receives free donor-recruitment ads, which appear as public service announcements on all the media from coast to coast. J. Walter Thompson, one of the world's largest advertising agencies, handles the Red Cross campaign without charge. For 1984, journalist Andrea Rock estimated the total value of such pro bono advertising services at $21.3 million.[39]

Despite these subsidies, Red Cross blood derivatives sold to hospitals and hemophiliacs are not substantially cheaper than those sold by commercial firms. A hemophiliac, whose life depends on adequate supplies of Factor VIII, may spend well over $50,000 a year for clotting factor alone. In other words, the Red Cross nonprofit Blood Services sells products it has had manufactured from freely donated plasma—and at a substantial profit.

In recent years, the American Red Cross has continued its policy of expansion and diversification, also venturing into the tissues and organs market. In 1984, the Red Cross board of governors, seeing "an opportunity for future growth," agreed to increase the organization's supply of tissues and organs. The rationale, as usual, was not lacking. "This is a very natural step for the Red Cross to take. Blood is technically a tissue too."[40] Accordingly, the American Red Cross Blood Services began a noncash transplant donation program at regional blood centers across the country, at the same time attempting to prevent remuneration of other tissue and organ suppliers. This provoked predictable hostility and started a series of turf battles with existing tissue banking organizations.

While the Red Cross entry into this field was in keeping with its

humanitarian tradition, the move was also consistent with its economic interest. In 1984 health insurers were paying out hundreds of
millions of dollars to organ suppliers, and demand was increasing.
Meanwhile the Red Cross blood program was reported to have
peaked, and the organization needed fresh markets and new sources
of revenue.[41]

There is nothing wrong with the Red Cross decision to engage in
commercial activities—providing it pays taxes when it competes with
other tax-paying organizations, does not seek a monopoly, and otherwise engages in "fair practices." It could even be argued that competition is good for the plasma or tissue banking industry and might
improve the general quality of its product. But by the same reasoning,
competition would also help patients who now receive all their blood
from the Red Cross without any real alternative. Competition on the
basis of the quality of the product—whether it is delivered by profit
or nonprofit organizations—can only be beneficial to the public.

It cannot be in the best interest of public health that a cartel of
nonprofit blood-collecting organizations should enjoy a near monopoly—and tax-exempt profits—with governmental support.[42] The fact
that these organizations bear almost no liability for the state of the
blood they supply is a questionable legal privilege. Until these blood
banking organizations are brought to stricter account, both financial
and legal, they will have little incentive to improve the quality of the
blood they provide to the American people. Even more significantly,
just as other participants in the health care industry are prevented
from making false claims regarding the safety of the products and
services they provide, the blood banking industry needs to be held to
a similar standard of honesty regarding the risks of the products and
services it provides.

4

The Blood Supply II:
The Plasma Sector
and the Role of the
Drug Companies

A great strength of the American system is that it has room for private enterprise and for the non-profit provision of human services. Sometimes the line between these functions becomes blurred.

Dr. Lewellys F. Barker, senior vice president of the American Red Cross, testifying at the 100th Congress

While tax-exempt organizations collect whole blood and blood components in the United States, a separate sector of the blood industry is responsible for the collection of plasma and its manufacture into blood derivatives.*

Controlled mainly by large pharmaceutical companies such as Armour, Cutter Laboratories, and Alpha Therapeutics, the plasma sector operates on an openly commercial, for-profit basis. In the past this has led to suspicion about profiteers trafficking in human blood and exploiting poor or underprivileged peoples. Yet ironically—and tragically—when AIDS first struck, the commercial sector acted more responsibly than the so-called nonprofits. Responding to consumer

---

*Whole blood is divided into *components*—primarily red cells, platelets, and plasma; plasma is further subdivided into multiple blood products called blood *derivatives*.

pressure—particularly from hemophiliacs, but also from European buyers—commercial plasma collectors took steps to safeguard their blood against AIDS in early 1983. By contrast the Red Cross, the AABB, and the CCBC initially denied that there was any significant connection between blood and AIDS and then, for two years, failed to take more stringent precautions to screen against the deadly disease.

A DUAL BLOOD SUPPLY SYSTEM

Over half of human blood volume consists of plasma, the fluid part of blood in which the cellular components are suspended. Composed mainly of water (90 percent) to facilitate transportation, plasma also contains many valuable proteins vital for clotting and fighting infections. We have already described Edward Cohn's new method—developed during World War II—of breaking down or fractionating plasma into vital blood derivatives like albumin, coagulation factors, and immunoglobulins. With the growing use of specific blood components, and the increasing demand for these therapeutic derivatives, fractionation has become the basis of a worldwide multibillion-dollar industry—not surprising since a fully processed unit of blood can eventually yield over $1000 worth of products.

Whole blood collections are geared towards ensuring an adequate supply of red cells, the mainstay of any blood transfusion system. But simply recovering plasma from whole blood is not sufficient to maintain enough plasma for use in derivatives. Fractionators require very large volumes of plasma to meet their manufacturing needs. For example, Factor VIII, used to treat hemophiliacs, is a blood plasma derivative in great demand. As a result, a separate blood plasma industry has arisen to fill the burgeoning demand for plasma derivatives. This industry is separate from the voluntary sector and very dependent on paid blood plasma donors. Unlike the standard blood donation, these donors have their blood removed and separated into red cells and plasma. The red cells are immediately transfused back into the patient while the plasma portion of the blood is retained for future use.

The plasma industry itself is a two-tiered system, consisting of plasmapheresis centers that collect blood plasma from paid donors, and pharmaceutical companies that fractionate this plasma and market it as separate derivative products manufactured from the blood

The Blood Supply II

plasma. These two activities have developed separately, though today about a third of U.S. plasma collection centers are owned by large fractionation companies.[1] Most of the remaining centers—over 300 are licensed to collect plasma in the U.S.—are owned by independent multilocation firms. These centers obtain blood plasma primarily from paid donors and contract to sell it to the pharmaceutical companies in bulk. There are a number of companies that buy and sell blood plasma within the United States and overseas, with some spot buying on the open market to accommodate seasonal fluctuations in demand.

A small but significant percentage of these blood plasma collection centers are run by community or Red Cross blood centers on a nonprofit basis. Again, this only means that blood *donors* are not paid for their plasma; the Red Cross is paid for the plasma, like any other commercial firm that collects blood plasma. A 1985 report by the Federal Office of Technology Assessment asserted: "Through its system of regional blood centers the Red Cross collects more plasma for fractionation than any other single entity in the world."[2]

Many American centers also sell their plasma to fractionators outside the United States in Europe, Japan, and South America. The United States is the international leader in blood plasma, collecting over 60 percent of the annual worldwide yield of 15 million liters and exporting several million liters to Japan and Europe.[3]

Blood plasma is collected through plasmapheresis, a process in which a person selectively donates only his plasma.* Although whole blood is drawn, the plasma is immediately separated out through centrifugation in a special instrument and then all the cells are transfused back, minus the plasma, through the same needle and tubing. The entire procedure takes about two and a half hour, although newly automated plasmapheresis equipment is available which can cut the time in half.

Since the body replenishes its plasma within days,† a person can

---

Hemapheresis is the general term for the technique whereby only a desired blood component is taken from the donor's blood and the remaining fluid and blood cells are immediately transfused back. This process helps alleviate the chronic shortage of donors by capitalizing on large, repeat collections from the same donors. The technique is increasingly common with platelets too.

†Although the fluid part of plasma regenerates within 24 hours, the regeneration of plasma proteins usually takes up to a week. Plasma collectors have been criticized for taking plasma at a rate which depletes plasma proteins and the valuable antibodies they contain.

donate plasma two times a week—as opposed to a maximum of five or six times a year for whole blood. (Red cells take two to six weeks to regenerate.) Another advantage is that more than twice the volume of blood plasma can be taken from a plasmapheresis donation than from the whole blood. In plasmapheresis, the plasma can also be frozen immediately and its proteins more effectively preserved.

Plasmapheresis donors are paid relatively little—between $5 and $20 for each donation. The fee varies to encourage more frequent donation: first-time donors and people who return within a week—or a month—are paid more; so are people who agree to get an injection for producing special antibodies.

Far fewer donors give plasma than whole blood but those who do so give on a regular basis, 35 times a year on average.* A fee is considered necessary since the procedure usually takes over two hours of a donor's time. A routine whole blood donation, by comparison, takes less than half an hour—but donors seldom repeat, with 1.5 donations a year being the average.[4] People with rare antibodies can give plasma more than 35 times annually and can thereby earn thousands of dollars a year.

There are two categories of plasma used in the commercial sector, "source" plasma and "recovered" plasma. Source plasma, the basis of the industry, is the raw material collected directly through plasmapheresis. It can also include whole blood donation if the plasma is removed and frozen immediately without preservatives: this is called fresh-frozen plasma.

Recovered plasma refers to what is salvaged after whole blood has outdated. Recovered plasma is considered inferior to source plasma and mainly used as a laboratory reagent to diagnose certain diseases. It is permitted for transfusion only when there is a shortage of source plasma. Nevertheless the demand for recovered plasma has been growing, and it provides an additional source of revenue for the Red Cross and other whole blood collectors. In the sixties when plastic collection bags made component separation a widespread practice— it became safer and easier to split blood up into specific components—organizations like the Red Cross were often left with surplus

---

*As of today there are no documented health problems with plasmapheresis donation. However, since the procedure became commonplace only in the 1970s—it began in the 1950s—some time will pass before all the potential long-term effects can be completely ruled out.[5] We know from experience with drug addicts that simply traumatizing one's vein with a large needle 35 times a year is unhealthy.

plasma collected from a given region.[6] In commercial fractionators like Armour and Hyland Therapeutics, they have found an important market for this component from their whole blood.

The centers that collect plasma today are, in part, an outgrowth of the commercial whole blood collectors of the past.[7] During the forties, these unlicensed commercial blood bank operators were allowed to provide blood only when there was a shortage that the voluntary organizations could not fill. Although officially discouraged, they continued to flourish through the sixties, when regulatory laws were lax and many prominent hospitals bought their blood. With no mechanism for oversight, a number of serious problems developed.

Later it was clearly demonstrated that some commercial establishments—particularly those buying blood in poverty-stricken areas—did not adequately screen their donors: they registered a significantly higher incidence of hepatitis than voluntary organizations.[8] The financial incentive to donate blood apparently led some underprivileged donors to misrepresent their state of health to commercial establishments. This finding led to the unfortunate stigmatization of all paid donor blood. While some commercial blood banks deserved to be put out of business, others tightened standards and improved services in accordance with the new regulations.

After Titmuss's influential book and the start of the National Blood Program in 1974, almost all American hospitals stopped buying blood from the discredited commercial banks. Forced out of the whole blood field, many commercial blood banks saw an opportunity in the expanding plasma sector. Therapeutic products processed from plasma were increasingly in need. Clinical use of blood derivatives was becoming widely accepted, and there was a huge demand for raw material. By the end of the seventies, commercial plasma collectors were supplying 4 million liters of plasma a year to fractionators. They were also beginning to exercise greater quality control, partly in response to the concerns of their customers, the pharmaceutical manufacturers.

Given the sensitive nature of their business, plasma collectors have often attracted adverse publicity. In 1976, a fire in Nicaragua destroyed one of the largest American plasma collection centers and created a public outcry against the practice of importing blood from developing countries.[9] The U.S. had been filling about 20 percent of its plasma needs from abroad, with the 150-bed plasmapheresis center in Nicaragua providing half of this foreign plasma. Now ethical questions were raised about exploiting poor, malnourished Third

World donors—taking too much blood and exposing them to infections*—as well as endangering Americans with questionable blood
from foreign sources.

With the loss of the Nicaragua center, American fractionators
began to acquire their own domestic plasma-collection facilities.
Major foreign plasma collection centers in Nicaragua, Haiti, and
Belize were all shut down. Today America is a major exporter, not an
importer, of blood plasma.

The plasma sector was also reputed to run fly-by-night collection
centers in skid-row neighborhoods where it exploited poor, inner-city
minorities—a perception strongly influenced by Titmuss's book.
Today many plasma centers are located in small urban and suburban
areas and around college campuses and shopping centers. However,
a small number of centers still collect plasma in prisons and from
Mexicans who enter the country illegally to sell their plasma along the
U.S.–Mexican border. This practice may soon be eliminated because
of greater safety standards demanded by the lucrative overseas markets. Statistically, most plasma donors are Caucasian and lower
working-class. Since money is the main incentive, donors often include temporarily laid-off workers and others seeking to supplement
their incomes. Blood plasma is screened and rejected if it does not
meet the specifications for laboratory tests established by the FDA.

It is a major misconception that almost all blood collected in the
United States comes from voluntary donors. In fact, a very significant
portion of blood collected in America is from paid donors. The issue
has been confused because of a general lack of understanding that
plasma is the major component of blood.

MANUFACTURING AND MARKETING PLASMA

Four pharmaceutical companies currently dominate the market for
plasma, manufacturing almost all blood derivatives used in the
United States. These four commercial fractionators, Hyland Therapeutics, Cutter Laboratories, Alpha Therapeutics, and Armour, are
themselves subsidiaries of four major corporations: Travenol, Bayer,
Green Cross, and Revlon, respectively. The New York Blood Center,

*Blood plasma contains the circulating antibodies used to fight infection.

a nonprofit blood bank, also owns a fractionation plant for its donors and for some Red Cross donors. Despite this corporate dominance, close to 20 percent of plasma derivatives sold in the United States are sold by the nonprofits—specifically the Red Cross and the New York Blood Center; as noted earlier, the sale of plasma derivatives puts the tax-exempt industry into direct competition with the commercial sector.

The United States is now the major world supplier of plasma products, both source plasma and plasma derivatives, and manufactures over 70 percent of the world's plasma products. While America has always been technologically advanced, there is another reason for its plasma dominance: the United States pays its plasma donors while many other countries expressly prohibit such payment. As a result several foreign countries, especially in Europe, are unable to meet their own plasma needs and depend on United States supplies.* Two of America's more economically aggressive and successful competitors, Germany and Japan, have secured their own supplies (Germany in 1977 and Japan in 1978) by buying U.S. fractionation plants which they now own through two of the big four, Bayer and Green Cross.

Since World War II, the most popular product of plasma fractionation—and the industry leader, usually accounting for 50 percent of sales—has been albumin. Albumin acts like a sponge to keep enough fluid in the blood vessels so the vessel walls will not collapse; and it is used to expand blood volume for shocks, burns, coronary bypass surgery, liver failure, and acute kidney disease.

Albumin is processed in two forms: normal serum albumin (NSA), which must have at least 96 percent albumin protein; and plasma protein fraction (PPF), which has a minimum of 85 percent albumin. Because it is cheaper to manufacture, PPF is preferred by most fractionators. Manufacturers and suppliers engage in annual bidding to set prices for albumin, and joint purchasing groups representing several hospitals can sometimes get a lower price for a large, reliable order. Nursing homes and dialysis centers often buy albumin locally on the spot market, since their needs are more irregular.

Guaranteeing a steady, reliable supply of albumin is important to hospitals because there is great volatility in the availability and prices

*By contrast, European countries collect more than enough whole blood to meet their own needs. They then export their surplus red cells to the United States under the trademark "Euroblood." New York, which lags behind other cities in blood self-sufficiency, imports as much as one third of its blood from Europe—predominantly from Switzerland, West Germany, and Belgium.[11]

of source plasma. It takes four to six months from collection to process plasma fully into a licensed, finished derivative. Meanwhile new shortages or surpluses can drastically affect the price. Manufacturers often move their product to different markets—or different countries, where they maintain alternate distribution networks—in order to take advantage of these sudden pricing shifts. This is a good example of how market forces may not only react to but even determine the availability of supplies. The product goes to the highest bidder.

Over the last decade and a half there has been some concern about the overuse of albumin.[12] Some countries, like Japan, have recently undertaken a concerted plan to reduce their consumption of albumin severely. My own experience suggests that there is more often an underuse of albumin. Patients who have blood loss and are transfused only with red cells are often missing albumin that they would have received had they been transfused with whole blood. Albumin is critically important in maintaining osmotic pressure within the blood vessel walls, and patients occasionally go into heart failure because of inadequate albumin levels. However in the last two years, as a result of various forces, the sale of albumin, once the industry pacesetter, has been overtaken by Factor VIII.

Coagulation factors—in particular antihemophilic factor (AHF), otherwise known as Factor VIII—are the other big sellers in the plasma market. AHF, a clotting factor required by hemophiliacs to stem bleeding, was first manufactured in 1966 and has seen the fastest growth of any plasma derivative. Today the sale of AHF, even more than that of albumin, drives the market and determines the profitability of the pharmaceutical companies.

AHF is an unstable protein and must be prepared as a powder and reconstituted with sterile water prior to injection. Factor IX complex is used for hemophilia B and for patients with inhibitors to Factor VIII. (Hemophilia B is a coagulation disorder very similar to hemophilia A except that Factor IX, as opposed to Factor VIII, is the missing clotting element. Approximately 13 percent of hemophiliacs in the United States have hemophilia B.)

Unlike other plasma derivatives, clotting factors must be made from plasma frozen immediately after withdrawal or else its activity or potency decreases. This makes it more difficult to treat Factor VIII against disease, though new virus sterilization processes have been developed. In the past, Factor VIII has been known to transmit hepatitis. During the AIDS crisis, it became especially menacing, since

Factor VIII is manufactured from batches of plasma pooled from hundreds, even thousands of donors.* A handful of AIDS patients who donated regularly—remember that 35 times is the *average*— could infect a whole year's supply.

This potential for disaster has already been realized; in fact, the National Hemophilia Foundation now confirms that half the hemophiliacs in the United States—about 10,000 people—are infected with the AIDS virus (HIV, or the human immune deficiency virus), which they contracted from Factor VIII, most before 1985. About fifteen percent of the spouses of HIV-infected hemophiliacs have also been infected with the AIDS virus.[13]

In the past four years, as concern about AIDS has intensified, AHF has been subjected to a variety of antiviral treatments. One inactivation process consists of adding an organic solvent and detergent to the Factor VIII.[14] Along with heat treatment, this method has resulted in a much lower infection rate. However, treatment also destroys about half of the Factor VIII, so that the yield is very low and more plasma is needed. As a result, there are now serious shortages of AHF and the price has shot up astronomically, from 50 to 800 percent per unit in the last two years alone.[15]

Altogether, the new, specially treated Factor VIII can now cost the average hemophiliac up to $70,000 a year, a prohibitive sum that has inflicted serious financial losses on many hemophiliacs, and put the latest, safest form of the product totally out of reach for others. Some hemophiliacs simply can't afford to buy Factor VIII that has been inactivated with the latest techniques; instead they must use the less safe product. One solution has been to offer the older Factor VIII for people already infected with HIV and to reserve the more expensive Factor VIII for those not yet exposed to the AIDS virus. Not surprisingly, this arrangement has come under criticism from many quarters—repeated exposure to HIV may hasten the onset of full-blown AIDS—yet it represents one effort at adapting to a growing, unmanageable crisis.[16]

A third plasma product, immune serum globulins, account for about 10 percent of plasma sales. Immune globulins produce antibodies to fight diseases like measles, mumps, tetanus, rabies, and hepatitis. Plasma is prepared from donors who have high globulin

---

*For economic reasons, plasma is pooled or mixed together before being fractionated. A single "pool" of plasma is normally made up of a thousand different donations, although in theory, Factor VIII could be processed from a single plasma unit.

levels—either naturally or induced—against a specific disease. Immune globulins are injected both intramuscularly and intravenously.
Inventories tend to run high and there are normally no problems
with supply.

Human plasma not acceptable for fractionation and injection is
used instead as a reagent for laboratory diagnostic studies, a growing
research field. While there is no danger of accidental transfusion,
some studies suggest that hospital workers may be at risk from
handling this material.

In addition to these known products, many new derivatives are
currently being explored. Proteins found in plasma are constantly
being investigated for therapeutic possibilities, and new AIDS antibodies are being sought. There are also new derivatives that have
appeared in Europe and await approval by the FDA.

Despite their questionable reputation, the commercial organizations in blood banking's plasma sector have performed an important
service. They have maintained an adequate supply of plasma and
plasma derivatives and they have done so at a reasonably high level of
quality. Although all paid blood seemed to be doomed in the early
1970s, the National Blood Policy has never moved to outlaw the
commercial plasma sector, as many thought it would. Meanwhile, it
has become clear that plasma collectors and pharmaceutical fractionators fulfill a vital need which the voluntary sector cannot meet. Paid
blood plasma donors are tolerated because it is the only way to keep
up with demand.

In 1979, the Red Cross—the only possible rival—did consider a
joint venture with Baxter-Travenol for a giant fractionation facility
that would have brought them 30 percent of the world plasma market.
But these plans were scrapped, owing as much to the negative public
relations effect as to the huge plant costs involved.

No new firm has entered the plasma sector in 15 years, and several
giants—Parke-Davis, Squibb, Upjohn, and Merck—have left. However, in addition to its plasma fractionation contract with Baxter-
Travenol in 1986, the American Red Cross announced a new alliance
with the corporate giant called the Value Management Relationship
(VMR). This alliance represents a useful combination of the nation's
two largest organizations involved in the blood industry, according to
the president of the American Red Cross, Richard Schubert: "The
VMR will enhance the premier position that each organization holds
in its respective product and service areas."[17] According to the congressional testimony of competitors like Alpha Therapeutics, however, the VMR will give the American Red Cross and Baxter-Travenol

unfair advantages and a near-monolithic dominance over the industry: "Their [the VMR's] ultimate and long-term calculation and effect will be to place the U.S. blood services complex in the hands of an alliance, or monopoly, composed of the not-for-profit ARC and the distinctly for-profit Baxter-Travenol."[18]

THE AIDS CRISIS: A DISTURBING TEST CASE

The behavior of the two blood industries during the AIDS crisis highlighted their differences and exposed a fundamental flaw in the system—specifically within the whole blood sector. While neither of the groups was particularly heroic, it was the voluntary, tax-exempt organizations—the Red Cross, the AABB, and the CCBC—who clearly evaded their responsibility to the public. Although this episode has been well documented elsewhere,[19] it bears retelling not only for the tragic past misconduct it reveals, but for the warning it implies for any similar crisis in the future.

In December 1982, the Centers for Disease Control (CDC) in Atlanta warned the blood industry of growing evidence that AIDS was caused by an infectious agent that had already begun to contaminate the nation's blood supply. For the first time, the CDC had documented AIDS cases in which the victims did not belong to any known high-risk group but at some point in the past had received a transfusion or used a blood-based product. It was a revelation with profound implications for the entire American public health system, yet the FDA took no immediate action.

A month later, in January 1983, the National Hemophilia Foundation asked blood and plasma collectors to screen all donors and to take steps to discourage AIDS high-risk groups from giving blood. Hemophiliacs are among the most vulnerable recipients of blood and the news had sent shock waves through this sizeable community.

The plasma sector, represented by the American Blood Resources Association (ABRA), immediately agreed to comply. Some commercial blood plasma purchasers did not even wait for the National Hemophilia Foundation to request the more exacting screening procedures. As early as December 1982, Armour began buying blood from low-risk suppliers and stopped buying it from high-risk areas like New York, San Francisco, and Los Angeles. Moreover, following the recommendations of January 1983, the commercial plasma sector as a whole instituted three separate procedures to screen donors. First, donors were questioned face to face and asked if they were either intravenous drug users or homosexuals. Next each donor was requested to sign an affidavit attesting to the veracity of his statement. Finally a physical examination of the lymph glands was conducted (lymphadenopathy was one of the earliest tests used to detect the presence of AIDS).

Meanwhile, the Red Cross and the other tax-exempt organizations refused to accept publicly the notion that AIDS could be transmitted through transfusion. They argued that the evidence remained "incomplete" and "inconclusive"[20] and they expressed concern about the adequacy of blood supplies, fearing that direct questioning might discourage donations. Fewer donations meant lower revenues and greater recruitment expenses. They also feared charges of invasion of privacy by homosexuals.[21] In sum, they discounted the CDC warning, ignored the recommendation from the National Hemophilia Foundation, and continued to accept blood from all donors. Over a year *after* the original CDC warning, Aaron Kellner, president of the New York Blood Center, said at a CCBC meeting in February 1984, "We're not convinced that AIDS is transmitted by blood transfusion. . . . The evidence is still very shaky."[22]

By March 1983, the U.S. Public Health Service had already announced that people in high-risk groups should not give blood; a few weeks later the FDA issued donor screening guidelines. These guidelines still fell short of those already adopted by the commercial plasma sector, which had to respond to its customers' concerns.

For the Red Cross and other tax-exempt organizations, the FDA recommended making educational material available to donors about AIDS high-risk groups. The FDA recommendations did not include a physical examination, direct questioning, or the signing of an affidavit. In the meantime, 1.5 million units of blood had been collected between January and March 1983, and no one will ever know how much contaminated blood slipped through because even these simple guidelines were not utilized.

By the middle of 1983, a Stanford blood banker, Dr. Edgar Engleman, realized that screening donors was not a strong enough precaution. He recommended screening blood as well. Since there was no test to detect AIDS yet—the virus had not been identified—Engleman chose a surrogate test that would detect a white cell abnormality frequently found in the blood of AIDS patients: the T-cell test.* If a donor's blood showed this T-cell abnormality, Engleman would as-

*T-cells are special white blood cells that produce antibodies to fight infection. A depleted or lowered T-cell count suggests the presence of the AIDS virus.

sume it was infected with AIDS and throw it out. If he was wrong, then the worst he had done was to waste a unit of blood; if right, as he frequently was, then he had protected his patients' lives. Engleman's screening was not as specific as an AIDS test but it was the next best thing.

In July Stanford became the first blood bank in the country to screen blood with the T-cell test. Despite an additional 10 percent surcharge, the test proved extremely popular with patients. Soon several other blood banks across the country instituted surrogate tests in order to remain competitive with Stanford. The core antibody test,* long debated for use against hepatitis, was now also adopted as a surrogate test for AIDS.

That summer, in an effort to publicize the growing problem, Engleman submitted an abstract to the annual meeting of the AABB. He urged the blood banking community to institute new blood tests against transfusion-transmitted AIDS and described his own efforts with the T-cell test. Five years later, testifying before the Presidential Commission on AIDS, Engleman described the reaction he received:

> Although we were disappointed that our abstract was rejected
> for presentation at the meeting, it was particularly distressing
> to discover later that the subject of transfusion-associated AIDS
> wasn't even on the meetings program. While we certainly don't
> believe there was a conscious conspiracy to repress information
> about transfusion-associated AIDS, there seemed to be great re-
> luctance among blood bankers to acknowledge the problem.[23]

In December 1983 the FDA recommended to the blood industry that it consider using the core antibody test as a surrogate test for AIDS. This was a relatively inexpensive and easy test to implement with existing blood bank equipment. However, the Red Cross and the AABB disapproved of the move, maintaining that nationwide surrogate testing was not necessary. Instead they pressured the FDA Blood Products Advisory Committee to avoid a decision and to appoint a task force to study the matter further.

In January of 1984, the *New England Journal of Medicine* published documentation of the first 18 transfusion-related AIDS tests. Despite

---

*The core antibody test detects antibodies to the core component of hepatitis B. According to a 1983 CDC study of AIDS patients, hepatitis B core antibodies were present in all intravenous drug users and in 88 percent of male homosexuals. By identifying and isolating the blood of these patients at high risk for AIDS, the core antibody test could have prevented some cases of transfusion-transmitted AIDS.

clear evidence that AIDS had been contracted as a direct result of blood or blood products, the Red Cross, the AABB, and the CCBC continued to refuse instituting the new tests, persisting in their claim that nationwide surrogate testing was unwarranted.[24]

Meanwhile, that spring, Dr. Engleman received an urgent phone call from a colleague hundreds of miles away. A patient with AIDS had confessed to donating blood at Stanford and other blood banks in the area. Engleman checked his records and found that the man's blood had tested abnormal and had been thrown out. Other blood banks in the area, who were not using any surrogate test for AIDS, did not fare so well. At least 11 known recipients had been transfused with contaminated blood from the same AIDS patient.[25]

In March 1984, the FDA task force met and the plasma industry declared that it would begin surrogate testing whether an agreement was reached or not. The commercial sector, under increasing pressure, felt it had to reassure its hemophiliac customers. By contrast, the Red Cross and the AABB still refused to comply. They claimed the test was not cost-effective and its reliability had still not been proved. Surrogate testing would compel them to throw out from 3 to 10 percent of their blood, and not all of it would be tainted by AIDS, forcing voluntary organizations to recruit more donors and so raise their expenses.

The voluntary, tax-exempt organizations maintained that present donor screening was adequate and safe. They agreed to do nothing, although they were worried by the split with the commercial sector, since they did not want to lose their important plasma market. It would hurt both their public image and sales if their standards were seen to be lax in comparison with the commercial collectors and their product were discredited. (It is important to remember that a great deal of effort had been expended to stigmatize the commercial collectors and their paid donors as providing an inferior blood product.)

When Margaret Heckler, then secretary of Health and Human Services, announced the discovery of the AIDS virus a month later, in April 1984, the Red Cross and the AABB were freed from the mounting pressure for surrogate testing. Heckler claimed that an AIDS test would be ready in six months and that it would be 100 percent safe. In fact, it took almost another year before testing for AIDS began in March of 1985. (Today there is still no direct, practical AIDS test).* In the interim, 10 million more units of untested blood were collected.

The entire episode shows the Red Cross Blood Services and the other tax-exempt organizations in an extremely damaging light. They initially resisted evidence linking AIDS and blood, publicly denying that a problem existed. Instead of alerting the public, they issued false assurances. They then opposed donor screening to discourage high-risk groups; and as the crisis intensified, they refused to test blood for close to two years, rejecting every form of surrogate testing and unnecessarily exposing the population to a greater risk of AIDS.

The final count is not in, but as of January 1990, the CDC estimates that 10,000 hemophiliacs—half of the entire American hemophiliac population—has been infected with AIDS. Another 12,000 people are believed to be HIV positive as a result of transfusion with tainted blood. The CDC estimates that of those who have not already died, the vast majority will develop full-blown AIDS within five to ten years of their transfusion. Hundreds, possibly thousands of spouses of those infected with the AIDS virus through contaminated blood have also been infected with the virus causing AIDS.

How many of these people might have been spared had the so-called nonprofit blood industry responded more quickly and appropriately to a national crisis?

The commercial plasma industry, because it is by its nature accountable to consumers, at least took some preliminary measures to safeguard the blood supply. To its credit, it began screening donors at high risk for AIDS two years before the so-called nonprofits. The voluntary, tax-exempt organizations, because they are not sufficiently accountable to anyone, failed to act in the best public interest. Their conduct during this period should put to rest once and for all the idea that because blood is collected by voluntary, tax-exempt organizations, these organizations will act in an altruistic way for the public good. It also raises an important question about their obligation to provide full disclosure about the safety of the blood supply.

---

*At the present time, it is still too difficult to perform a test that can directly detect the presence of the AIDS virus except in special research laboratories. A virus is usually more difficult to detect than antibodies that form in response to the virus.

5

The Risks
of Transfusion Today

Human blood has always been and always will be the world's most
dangerous drug. The lengthening list of transfusion-transmitted
microorganisms includes syphilis; malaria; hepatitis B;
cytomegalovirus; non-A, non-B hepatitis; Epstein-Barr; HIV; and now
HTLV-I. No one seriously doubts that others will follow, *ad infinitum.*

> *Dr. Thomas Asher, testifying before the Presidential Commission
> on the HIV Epidemic, May 9, 1988*

The person about to have a blood transfusion today confronts
many risks. Some are life-threatening, while others are mild and
relatively minor. But almost all are unnecessary and avoidable.

Perhaps the biggest problem is the lack of information—or the
misinformation—that passes for accepted wisdom. The risk of AIDS
from a blood transfusion, for example, may be significantly higher
than most published statistics suggest. The risk of hepatitis is much
higher, and the disease kills more people than does even AIDS. It is
worth noting that it is only recently, with a new test for hepatitis "C"
reportedly developed, that blood banking organizations have openly
acknowledged the full extent of hepatitis infection in the blood supply.[1]

One of the primary purposes of this book is to enable members of
the public to understand for themselves what the real risks of transfusion are. At a time when society as a whole is beset by an increasingly
politicized public health debate, and when the facts about transfusion

71

are frequently distorted, it is important for each individual to know as much as possible in order to make informed and responsible choices.

THE RISKS OF TRANSFUSION: AN OVERVIEW

Blood transfusion is a lifesaving measure but it also carries many risks and hazards. Receiving foreign blood from several anonymous sources—the average transfusion consists of 5.4 components—poses manifold threats to the human body. For the sake of convenience, the risks associated with transfusion therapy today can be classified as infectious and noninfectious complications.

Infectious complications result from the transmission of disease agents through the blood. In 1943, P. B. Beeson first reported that patients developed jaundice a few months after transfusion.[2] Beeson identified blood as the vehicle for infectious transmission. Since then, the number of diseases known to spread through the blood has grown and multiplied. Today, infections that can be transmitted through blood transfusions include: non-A, non-B hepatitis; hepatitis B; AIDS; cytomegalovirus infection; Epstein-Barr virus; HTLV-I; HTLV-II; syphilis; and malaria. Other rare infectious complications are: HIV-2; Chagas' disease; brucella abortus; salmonella septicaemia; SPLV or B-19 virus; toxoplasma gondii; and babesia microti.

In July 1988, researchers at Yale School of Medicine raised the possibility that some cases of Alzheimer's disease may be caused by viral infection.[3] Human white blood cells from people with Alzheimer's disease and their relatives were injected into the brain of hamsters and produced brain deterioration. However, the Yale scientists emphasized that their conclusions were tentative and required further study.

In July 1989, experts became concerned that Lyme disease could be spread through blood transfusions. Lyme disease is caused by an infectious agent, a bacterium related to the one that causes syphilis—a disease that is spread through transfusions. French and American researchers have already proven the durability of the Lyme spirochete by keeping it alive for six weeks in conditions akin to the storage of blood.[4] At the present time, however, blood banks do not test for the presence of the Lyme spirochete, and they do accept donors who have had Lyme disease in the past.

Without formal epidemiological and laboratory studies, critics contend that the absence of Lyme disease cases associated with transfusions offers a false sense of security. Many transfusion recipients die from their underlying disease before Lyme has time to develop. The low rate of detection of the Lyme spirochete in the blood may simply reflect an inability to isolate the organism with current techniques. Further research and close medical surveillance are needed to follow individuals who received blood from donors testing positive for Lyme disease. It is important to determine the frequency with which healthy carriers spread the Lyme spirochete in transfusions.

In addition to the above infections or contagious diseases there are a group of noninfectious complications resulting from transfusion that are known as immunologic reactions.

The body has a highly specialized immune system that provides a basic defense against any foreign substance entering the blood. This system is so sensitive that it recognizes an intrusion by any agent not intrinsic to the body itself. In transfusion, immunologic reactions occur because of the extraordinary degree of variability between the blood constituents or substances of any two individuals, differences that can set off an immune response. In fact, the chances of getting an exact match of all the blood components in transfusion is less than one in 100,000.* As a result of such specificity, the immune system of a recipient can turn against the blood of a donor, treating it as a foreign invading agent.

Immune reactions may be either immediate, occurring during transfusion, or delayed (usually between a week to ten days). They vary in severity from the trivial, such as hives, to the life threatening, such as anaphylaxis, which involves the complete collapse of the circulation. A mismatch of the major blood types—for instance, giving type A blood to a type B patient—results in such complete clotting and destruction of the blood (known as severe hemolytic reaction) that death is a frequent occurrence.

HEPATITIS

The most common infection transmitted by blood is caused by any one of a dozen viruses that can invade and infect the liver, resulting in a condition known as hepatitis, or inflammatory liver disease. Approximately one out of every ten individuals who receives a blood transfusion will contract hepatitis.

*The individuality of the more than 600 blood subtypes is so distinct that blood has long been the standard measure for paternity testing. It is accepted as legal proof in a court of law.

The liver is responsible for the transformation of most of the food we eat into fats or sugars. These materials are then either stored or used up by the body. The liver is also a major organ for the elimination of waste products. It detoxifies potential poisons by combining them with special substances that makes these products water soluble and ready for excretion by the kidneys into the urine. The liver performs many other biochemical reactions upon which life depends.

An individual can tolerate up to 75 percent destruction of the liver by disease and still survive. Beyond that level, loss of life is likely to occur. People whose livers are destroyed may turn yellow or become jaundiced. The yellow coloration occurs because bile pigments, normally transformed in the liver so they can be excreted through the urine, are not chemically altered in the damaged liver. Instead, the bile pigments pile up in the body.

These bile pigments, which give our urine its yellow color, will cause the individual himself to turn yellow or jaundiced when they are not properly eliminated. In jaundice, the brownish urine is often accompanied by a disagreeable odor. The skin is itchy, due to retention of bile salts.

However, the liver is a resilient organ and infections that cause only partial damage, say 10 to 15 percent, will engender no visible change in most people. Approximately 10 to 15 liver tests have been developed in the past 20 years that can be performed by analyzing a sample of a patient's blood. These tests reveal inflammation and damage that would otherwise go unnoticed and, in earlier days, would have remained undetected.

The liver normally produces minimal pain even when injured or inflamed because it has few pain fibers. In the initial phase of hepatitis, the liver cells, of which there are billions, become mildly damaged and the organ becomes inflamed. In most cases, the individual is unaware of the disease.

The first sign of liver disease is the yellowish color appearing on the surface of the skin and in the eyes. The development of tests capable of detecting subtle levels of damage led to the discovery that most individuals whose liver is invaded by a hepatitis virus appear only mildly ill. In some cases they may not realize they're sick at all, or they may feel only slightly fatigued.

Only between 5 and 10 percent of individuals who become infected with a viral hepatitis will develop jaundice. In other words, unless the appropriate tests are undertaken, the overwhelming majority of individuals who contact hepatitis will remain unaware of it. They may feel mildly unwell but will have no outward manifestation of the disease.

When the liver is invaded in this way, the body responds by making antibodies in an attempt to neutralize or kill the invading virus. In approximately 50 percent of such cases, the virus is completely elimi- nated and becomes undetectable. Sometimes the only signs that an individual has been infected are the antibodies that remain in the blood and protect that person from future infections. These individ- uals are no longer contagious.

In recent years, some of the 10 to 12 viruses known to cause hepati- tis have become better understood. There are three major varieties of acute hepatitis that we can identify.*

Hepatitis A is usually mild and rarely associated with transfusions. The carrier state is not prolonged but it can cause jaundice and can be transmitted by blood transfusions. Blood is not tested for hepatitis A because of cost considerations and because most individuals who become infected do not become chronic carriers.

Hepatitis B is the most common form of hepatitis worldwide and is a known potential killer. In 1983, the World Health Organization estimated that there were 200 million carriers of hepatitis B in the world—or about 5 percent of the earth's human population.[5] Hepati- tis B is especially widespread in Southeast Asia and tropical Africa. In contrast to hepatitis A, the high rate of infection for hepatitis B occurs because people infected with hepatitis B become chronic car- riers capable of infecting other people for many years, particularly through intimate contact such as blood transfusion.

In the United States, 4.2 percent of the population, or about 9 million people, are hepatitis B carriers, and in some areas, the inci- dence is considerably higher.[6] The number of new U.S. cases has risen dramatically in the last decade, from about 200,000 a year in 1978 to 300,000 new cases a year today.[7] Among Asian immigrants into the United States the rate of previous hepatitis infection is in excess of 50 percent.[8]

Like AIDS, hepatitis B is a sexually transmitted disease; and like AIDS, hepatitis B spreads easily through blood. Those at highest risk for hepatitis B infection are intravenous drug users, homosexual men

*Another form of hepatitis can also be contacted by chemical poisons, of which alcohol is the most common example. Chemical hepatitis, which can also be caused by certain medications, is one of the few forms of hepatitis that cannot be transmitted by a blood transfusion.

with multiple sex partners, those who live with a carrier, and immigrants from areas with a high rate of infection. In addition, all operating room personnel, dentists, and health care workers who have frequent exposure to blood are at high risk for this disease. A National Institutes of Health study in 1986 reported that among anesthesiologists in practice for several years, the incidence of hepatitis B is 43 percent.[9] The CDC estimates that 12,000 health care workers a year become infected with hepatitis B. About 500 to 600 of these will require hospitalization and 700 to 1200 will become HBV carriers. Approximately 250 health care workers each year will die from their infection with hepatitis B.[10] The virus can enter the body via cuts, scratches, and accidental needle pricks, as well as toothbrushes and razor blades.

In 1976, Baruch S. Blumberg won a Nobel Prize for his discovery and work with the hepatitis B surface antigen.* Blumberg had made his discovery in 1963 and called it the Australia antigen. In 1966, he realized it was, in fact, the antigen for hepatitis B. It took six more years to develop a screening test for hepatitis B and three additional years before the FDA, in 1975, officially adopted the hepatitis B test for all donor blood. This lag is not untypical of the long process involved in implementing changes to the management of the nation's blood supply, which persists to this day.

Blumberg's test for hepatitis B surface antigens, which is basically a test for virus particles, has helped considerably to reduce the rate of transfusion-associated hepatitis B. On the other hand, it has not been eliminated because the test will not detect all carriers. As a result hepatitis B still accounts for about 10 percent of the nation's transfusion-related hepatitis cases, or at least 25,000 people a year.[11]

Clinical features of hepatitis B range from totally asymptomatic cases with minimal fatigue and relatively low-grade fever to cases with loss of appetite and jaundice. The most severe infections can lead to mental confusion, hemorrhaging, severe anorexia, and vomiting: the majority of these patients usually die within 30 to 90 days.

Chronic active hepatitis, which occurs in 5 to 10 percent of hepatitis B cases, is a slowly progressive form of the disease that may lead to liver failure over a period of many months or years. The progression of this form of hepatitis is variable, though ultimately such impair-

---

*An antigen is a molecule that causes the formation of an antibody. Surface antigen refers to the fact that the antigen is found on the surface of the cell.

ment of liver function can lead to death. An estimated 5 to 15 percent of chronic hepatitis B victims slowly develop cirrhosis and liver failure. However, most cases of transfusion-hepatitis death occur a long time after the initial transfusion and so these deaths are often not reported as being due to a blood transfusion. This omission leads to significant underreporting of transfusion death.

The CDC now recommends screening all pregnant women for hepatitis B. Mothers who are carriers may have no symptoms but their babies have an 80 percent chance of acquiring the infection. According to the CDC, almost 90 percent of infected infants—about 3,500 babies a year—become carriers. Of these, at least 25 percent—or over 850 babies a year—will die from cirrhosis of the liver or liver cancer.[12]

In many parts of the world, there is strong evidence of a link between chronic hepatitis due to the B virus and the occurrence of liver cancer. And the relationship between chronic hepatitis B infection and the occurrence of a number of immune complex disorders is now recognized.[13] Like the AIDS virus, with which it shares several similarities, the hepatitis B virus damages the general immunity of the patient and thus makes him vulnerable to other diseases. The virus can also cause the body to attack itself, as in polyarteritis nodosa, when the nerve sheets are attacked by the body's own immune system after being triggered by the hepatitis B virus.

A patient whom I recently saw in consultation received a blood transfusion during surgery which transmitted hepatitis B. This woman developed polyarteritis nodosa triggered by the immune complexes in hepatitis B. My patient was left with her arms and legs semiparalyzed. She does not have the use of her hands and must wear splints and braces on all four limbs. This woman, who was not advised about the risks of transfusion nor the possibility of postponing surgery so she could store her own blood, is now suing the hospital and the physicians who treated her for failing to inform her of safer alternatives to standard blood transfusion. Like her, most transfusion recipients are not aware, nor are they informed, that they have a 5 to 10 percent chance of contracting an infection from their blood transfusion.

After Blumberg's discovery of the hepatitis B antigen in the 1960s, and the exclusion of paid donors by blood banks, most experts believed that the plague of hepatitis had been contained. This view proved totally unfounded. It soon became clear that, in addition to types A and B, there were other unidentified viruses capable of causing the hepatitis syndrome and destroying the liver.

One of the more unusual agents that causes hepatitis is the hepatitis delta virus. This virus is not screened for by any blood bank although such a screening test exists. Infection with delta hepatitis causes no obvious physical change in the liver. However, when an individual becomes infected with both hepatitis B and delta hepatitis, the two viruses acting together attack the liver in a devastating way. Death within 90 days is far more likely than after infection with the hepatitis B virus alone. Many individuals who have been infected with either delta hepatitis or hepatitis B are unaware of the disastrous risks they face should they become infected with a second virus.

In addition to these, there are still multiple viruses—the exact number is unknown—that can cause severe hepatitis and for which there is no existing test. The disease caused by this group of viruses is called non-A, non-B hepatitis (NANB), simply because it does not fit into any of the other major categories. The overwhelming majority of transfusion-associated hepatitis cases—90 percent, or about a quarter of a million people in the United States each year—become infected with non-A, non-B hepatitis from a blood transfusion. In other words, 7 to 10 percent of all transfusion recipients in the United States develop hepatitis non-A, non-B. This is, or should be, a very sobering statistic. The figures worldwide range from a low of 2 percent in Australia to 44 percent in Japan.[14]

Many individuals who appear completely healthy are carriers of various viruses which can lead to slow, progressive destruction of the liver. When liver cells are inflamed and damaged they may lose some of their function. If they are damaged severely enough, these cells die. When large numbers of liver cells die, scar tissue forms. If the cells of the liver become extensively replaced by scar tissue, the resulting condition is called cirrhosis.

Cirrhosis is a chronic liver disease that is irreversible. It occurs in 15 percent of non-A, non-B cases—or in 0.3–0.4 percent of all transfusion recipients.[15] Other estimates place a patient's chance of developing cirrhosis from a blood transfusion as 1 in 200, even with the new surrogate or indirect tests.[16]

Based on several studies and statistics supplied by the U.S. Public Health Service,[17] anywhere from 10,000 to 15,000 Americans each year will develop cirrhosis and eventually die from the disease. However, unless a special note is made on the death certificate that the cirrhosis was related to hepatitis, which in turn was related to a transfusion, no causal connection will be established.

Most people are familiar with cirrhosis in connection with alcohol abuse. Alcohol is toxic to the liver. When consumed in large quantities on a continuing basis for many years, it eventually destroys the liver and kills the patient. Similarly, depending on the natural immunity of a given individual, hepatitis may destroy a person's liver in three months; or it may be a very slow, progressive disease that destroys the liver over a period of 5, 10, or occasionally even 20 to 30 years. The end result, however, is frequently death, although some individuals with severe liver damage may succumb to another affliction such as heart disease, before the liver fails completely. This is another reason why the impact of hepatitis is underappreciated.

Death from cirrhosis of the liver is a painful, wasting condition. The individual loses weight because he becomes unable to eat and digest his food. The body becomes progressively yellow and the abdomen swollen with fluid as the victim shrinks down and consumes his own muscles. Such a person, in effect, dies from starvation, despite the presence of food. Even intravenous feeding will not help such patients because the liver is essential for the metabolism of the nutrients provided by the intravenous infusion. Victims of cirrhosis die from an accumulation of waste products and starvation because they are unable to metabolize the food they are given.

Hepatitis manifests itself in a highly variable manner, ranging from a mild infection with complete recovery to an infected carrier state with no obvious disease. At the other end of the spectrum, it infects individuals who are superficially healthy but who actually harbor a significant disease slowly destroying their liver. Hepatitis, in its multiple forms, remains a serious threat to public health.

Historically it has always been difficult to ascertain the full extent of hepatitis in any given population, and the chances of becoming seriously infected. Many cases still remain undetected. Others are unreported. The official estimates by the Centers for Disease Control—the organization is charged by the federal government with tracking nationwide hepatitis—are hampered by widespread underreporting. Some hospitals have even been accused of a reluctance to report hepatitis cases out of fear for their own reputation.[18]

One reason why most cases of posttransfusion hepatitis are unreported is that no one runs the appropriate tests on patients 30 to 90 days after transfusion, once they have left the hospital. Two new surrogate tests, the alanine aminotransferase (ALT) and the core-antibody B tests, have reduced hepatitis infections in the blood supply, but claims of their effectiveness have been exaggerated and remain unsubstantiated by any reliable study.

It must be remembered that these are indirect tests: one of them, the core-antibody B, is simply another test for hepatitis B, already being screened for by the hepatitis B surface antigen test. Some hard follow-up evidence is needed to define the reduction in the incidence of hepatitis that has occurred as a result of these tests.

Today hepatitis remains the single greatest risk for patients facing a blood transfusion. Thousands of blood recipients will die this year as a result of a hepatitis infection leading to cirrhosis. Tens of thousands are infected now and over a hundred thousand will ultimately develop nonfatal complications that may incapacitate them for months or even shorten their lifespan in some cases.

At the present time, only the hepatitis B virus is routinely screened for by a blood test.* There is no screening for hepatitis A or delta hepatitis. Blood banks now perform other, indirect liver tests that can at least detect the presence of liver damage and eliminate some carriers. However, despite these advances, the best estimate by the American Red Cross is that 5 percent of those who receive a transfusion contract hepatitis, and the more realistic figure is probably closer to 10 percent. Even with the lower 5 percent estimate, we are left with 200,000 cases of transfusion hepatitis each year. As of today, there are still no cures and no effective treatment for this widespread, potentially fatal blood-borne disease.

NEW HEPATITIS "C" TEST

In April 1989, the Chiron Corporation announced a new screening test that identifies blood tainted with non-A, non-B hepatitis.[19] The test, the first of its kind, is being hailed as a major breakthrough. If it lives up to its billing, the new test could cause a significant reduction in the numbers of people infected with viral hepatitis through a blood transfusion and this advance would be a genuine cause for celebration. However, given what we know about hepatitis and the history of blood banking, a word of caution is in order.

The new Chiron test only detects one of the viruses that causes hepatitis non-A, non-B, a virus tentatively called virus "C." There are many viruses that attack the liver—remember that hepatitis non-A, non-B refers to an unknown number of multiple organisms—and it

*A few blood banks do conduct an entire battery of liver tests. However, the majority do not perform such tests because they have not been officially recommended. It is the author's opinion that any individual who exhibits liver damage should be suspect as a possible carrier of one form or another of hepatitis (see next chapter).

remains to be seen whether this new, previously unidentified virus "C" is the cause of a significant amount of non-A, non-B hepatitis. The new test will have to be implemented and studied for several years before any conclusions can be drawn. Dr. Jerome Zeldis of the University of California at Davis, a hepatitis researcher and physician, explained the situation:

> I think it's going to take at least a few years before we actually understand the life cycle of this virus and how it can be manifested and how we can best diagnose it. The best example of this would be hepatitis B, where it took us another seven years to figure out all the different antigens and markers for this infection.[20]

Hopefully the new test will create a significant reduction in exposure to hepatitis, but the exact amount remains to be proven by careful analysis and research. The Chiron claims of 80 to 100 percent accuracy do not seem realistic,[21] especially in light of previous safety claims by the blood banking establishment. In 1975, after implementing the hepatitis B test, blood bankers made similar claims about ridding the nation's blood supply of all hepatitis. After the continued occurrence of thousands of new hepatitis cases, they realized that they had identified only one virus. A similar situation could exist once the hepatitis "C" test is further defined—it may only eliminate a limited number of hepatitis cases and leave many other viruses that cause the disease at large.

The Chiron scientists acknowledged that they had never succeeded in isolating or seeing the new hepatitis "C" virus; rather, using ingenious molecular biology techniques, they were able to develop a test that identifies antibodies to the virus. This antibody-identification technique has certain limitations. Hepatitis B, for example, has multiple antibodies, some of which are not helpful in identifying the carrier state in healthy donors. Similarly, the Chiron test was developed from people who were diseased, and may not prove useful in identifying healthy donors who are carriers.

To date, the new hepatitis C test appears to be nonspecific, so that a significant number of false positives are showing up. Another drawback is that there is no second, confirmatory test to verify the original result.

While one can only applaud the efforts of the Chiron scientists and hope that their optimistic claims will be validated, as of today the nation's blood supply remains dangerously threatened by hepatitis.

The average patient receiving a blood transfusion still faces a 1 in 10 chance of infection. Preliminary results indicate that the new test may, at best, reduce this number to 1 in 20. After they had offered a tentative cure for the hepatitis problem, blood bankers were more open than usual in admitting the extent of the danger: they acknowledged that anywhere from 150,000 to 200,000 people contract hepatitis non-A, non-B each year from a blood transfusion;[22] and of these, about 15,000 people per year may develop severe or fatal liver disease.[23] Until we have any proof to the contrary, these figures must remain a fair and accurate warning to anyone contemplating a transfusion from the national blood supply.

CYTOMEGALOVIRUS

Cytomegalovirus or CMV is a herpes virus that can lead to serious disease in compromised hosts. An opportunistic organism,* CMV is especially dangerous to infants and immunosuppressed patients. With the spread of AIDS, the growing use of transplants, and new treatments like chemotherapy, the number of patients with decreased immunity—hence the number of those susceptible to CMV—has risen significantly.

Infection with CMV is very common but generally asymptomatic. It is estimated that more than 50 percent of adults in the industrialized world have been infected with CMV—and the figure is much higher in underdeveloped areas.[24] Many of these infections are secondary or latent—latent infections are hidden infections kept in check by a healthy body—but they can be reactivated, even in the presence of antibodies. In healthy individuals with a latent infection, small amounts of the virus are intermittently produced, but they are rendered innocuous by an intact immune system. Active infection only occurs when enough of the virus is produced to overcome this immunity and spread to other cells.

CMV is considered one of the infectious agents most frequently transmitted by transfusion. The latent virus often lives in the white cells and so can be transmitted directly through the blood. A donor who tests positive for CMV may be infectious, even if no active infec-

---

*An opportunistic organism is an organism that would normally not be capable of causing infection in a healthy person but can cause serious injury in a person whose immunity is compromised.

tion is present. The proportion of units that transmit the virus, roughly between 3 and 12 percent, is higher than the prevalence of active infection within the population, which is 2 to 3 percent.[25] These figures strongly suggest that CMV is transmitted through blood as a latent virus by many individuals who are actually healthy carriers.

In data pooled from 15 studies in 1984, the rate of CMV infection through blood transfusion was 13.5 percent. This would suggest that up to half a million Americans each year may be infected with CMV through blood transfusions. Recently, with the advent of AIDS, the incidence of CMV has reportedly been higher.

Fortunately, most cases of CMV are relatively mild. However, since infection with this virus is not tested for after transfusion, we do not know how many patients have a difficult course recovering from their disease due to complications from undetected CMV infection, rather than from their underlying illness.

The risk of contracting CMV through a blood transfusion was not reported until 1966, when two patients developed mononucleosis after open-heart surgery. The risk of viral transmission appears to be related to the amount of blood transfused: the more units of blood, the higher the risk of infection. However, blood that has been frozen and stored in glycerol does not transmit the virus after it is reconstituted.[26] Leukocyte or white blood concentrates carry the highest risk of infection.

Since most causes of CMV are not symptomatic, blood bankers have made little effort to minimize this risk of transmission through blood. However, there is a growing number of people for whom CMV poses a serious threat. According to a recent study, the known groups of patients at risk of opportunistic infection with CMV include "pregnant women; premature babies; patients treated by transplantation; patients treated with intensive chemotherapy for malignancy; patients immunosuppressed for other reasons; patients with diseases leading to cellular immunodeficiency including AIDS; splenectomized patients."[27]

When CMV appears in healthy individuals, it manifests itself as a form of mononucleosis, with fever and headache. However, there is rarely tonsillitis or pharyngitis, as there is in the mononucleosis connected with Epstein-Barr virus. Pneumonia and myocarditis can also occur. The disease lasts between two and four weeks and is self-limiting.

People with impaired immunity, either from disease or drugs, are much more susceptible to CMV infection and in these cases the virus can lead to severe illness and death. It is important to realize that, as in hepatitis, the immune state of an individual at the time of infection is critical in determining the response to the virus—and therefore how sick he or she will become. Thus one catches a cold when one goes out poorly dressed in freezing weather. The so-called "cold" does not occur directly because of the weather. Rather, it occurs because exposure to the cold lowers one's immunity so that a virus or other infectious organism already present in the body can spread rapidly.

Performing surgery on a patient who has a cold (that is, lower immunity) can have serious consequences. Blood loss alone, or any surgery, will also markedly compromise a patient's immunity. Recent experiments with animals at the Yale School of Medicine have shown that simple hemorrhage, without major tissue trauma, can depress the immune system and enhance susceptibility to infection.[28]

With regard to CMV, most people will have a relatively mild illness because their immune system is intact at the time of infection. However, if there is significant blood loss due to medical or surgical procedure, immunity will be compromised. As a result, a transfusion with CMV virus will lead to significant illness, including the development of hepatitis, since the virus can multiply rapidly.

Most patients show active CMV infection after organ transplants. Bone marrow transplant recipients are particularly vulnerable to serious CMV infection. CMV causes more deaths, especially from pneumonia, than any other agent in bone marrow transplants. Kidney, heart, and heart-lung transplant patients are also extremely susceptible for CMV. Autopsies have shown that even when it kills, CMV infection is often asymptomatic.[29] As a result, death from this cause is still underreported.

A mother infected with active CMV has a 30 to 40 percent chance of transmitting the virus to the fetus. In 5 to 10 percent of these cases, the infant will be born mentally retarded or with a serious hearing loss. In premature babies whose birthweight is below 3.2 pounds and whose mother lacks antibodies to CMV, there is a 25 to 30 percent chance of contracting the virus. One quarter of these infants will die.[30]

Altogether, CMV is the most common cause of congenital infection. In 1980, Dr. Edgar Engleman and his colleagues at Stanford devised a a simple blood test to detect the presence of antibodies to CMV. Engleman demonstrated that by using only CMV seronegative blood, the deadly effects of transfusion-transmitted CMV in premature infants could be completely avoided. Testifying before the Presidential Commission on AIDS in 1988, Engleman described the reaction his test received from the blood banking establishment:

> The cost of the test was no more than $2.00 and the results, which were published in peer-reviewed medical journals, were clear cut. Did the blood banking organizations adopt the test to protect susceptible patient groups?
>
> For the first 5 years after the results were published the AABB and the Red Cross did not endorse CMV testing, and many blood bankers called such testing impractical or inexact, a theme we heard again with the AIDS surrogate screening. Even now, the AABB Standards for Blood Banks and Transfusion Services call for blood banks to perform CMV testing only "where transfusion-associated CMV disease is a problem." Note that in contrast to the AIDS epidemic where we were forced to rely on indirect tests until 1985, when it came to CMV we had an inexpensive and highly specific test as well as hard evidence that by using the test in well-defined clinical situations, substantial morbidity and mortality could be avoided.[31]

Engleman's testimony suggests that blood recipients should be tested for CMV prior to transfusion. If a recipient is negative for CMV, he should not be transfused with blood from donors who are chronic carriers of the virus. In the case of people who have been previously exposed to CMV, the state of the blood donor's CMV infectiousness would not be relevant. Of course, such an effort would involve the introduction of an additional test.

Engleman's experience with the CMV test highlights the blood industry's innate conservatism and resistance to change. It also suggests, as some critics have alleged, that blood banks are more concerned with transfusion injuries that are immediate and lethal—and thus less expensive to trace—than with injuries that are delayed and less clearly visible.[32]

CMV is found not only in blood, but in saliva, urine, cervical secretions, and breast milk. The percentage of the population infected rises steadily from birth, with about 5 percent infected, to a plateau at age 30 of about 54 percent.[33]

Sexual transmission is also an important route for CMV, which is officially classified as a "sexually transmitted disease" (STD). The virus has been linked to Kaposi's sarcoma, a tumor associated with AIDS. Homosexuals with AIDS have a far higher rate of CMV infection than hemophiliacs and others who have contracted the disease through nonsexual means. Active homosexuals are almost invariably and repeatedly infected with CMV. High CMV infection rates have also been registered among promiscuous women.

Without referring to the blood supply, the Centers for Disease Control estimates that there will be one million new cases of CMV in the United States next year. Such a dramatic surge in the general population will certainly translate into increased risk for transfusion recipients.

EPSTEIN-BARR VIRUS

Like CMV, Epstein-Barr virus (EBV) is a herpes virus found throughout the world. EBV often manifests itself as mononucleosis. Known as "the kissing disease," the Epstein-Barr virus is most often transmitted through saliva. However, chronically transfused patients, such as hemophiliacs, have a high rate of EBV infection. So do homosexuals and other groups at high risk for AIDS. EBV has also been reported for patients transfused for cardiac bypass surgery and for splenectomy.

Children are more susceptible to EBV than any other group. In poor and underdeveloped nations, they contract EBV by the age of five, when it manifests as an acute viral illness. In more affluent nations like the United States, Epstein-Barr appears as infectious mononucleosis and hits teenagers and young adults. Fever, profound malaise, pharyngitis, and lymphadenopathy are frequent symptoms. In people over 30 and the elderly, EBV can result in atypical glandular fever.

Infectious mononucleosis from a blood transfusion usually occurs in recipients 21 to 30 days after they have been transfused. Most patients recover within a few weeks, but it sometimes takes much longer to recuperate. Since there is no known specific therapy for the disease, this period can be uncomfortably protracted. A chronic or recurrent syndrome associated with infectious mononucleosis can appear. Often this recurrence is connected to physical and emotional stress or to another viral infection. Due to the absence of any known treatment, psychological support is often recommended to help the patient in his or her convalescence.

More than 90 percent of blood donors normally have neutralizing antibodies to EBV that coexist with the latent virus. As a result, if more than one unit of blood is transfused, the chances are that one of the units will already have antibodies to EBV that neutralize the infection. While EBV via transfusion is relatively uncommon, it can be devastating when transmitted to immune-compromised patients not previously infected. Today posttransfusion EBV has increased and, under certain circumstances, it has even been identified with some forms of cancer.[34]

HUMAN T-CELL LYMPHOTROPIC VIRUS-I

Human T-cell lymphotropic virus-I (HTLV-I) belongs, like the AIDS virus, to the family of retroviruses.* HTLV-I was first identified by Dr. Robert C. Gallo of the National Cancer Institute in 1981. It has since been shown to be transmissible via transfusion. Like AIDS, the disease is believed to spread through sexual contact, blood, shared needles, and from mother to infant. In Japan, where families have been followed for a decade or more, HTLV-I has been found to spread over a period of years through nonsexual contact with various members of the family.

A potentially lethal virus, HTLV-I may cause a fatal form of leukemia called adult T-cell leukemia/lymphoma, which is a cancer of the blood-forming system: HTLV-I may also cause a severe neurological disorder called tropical spastic paraparesis, which resembles multiple sclerosis. Infections with HTLV-I may be latent for up to 20 years.

Infections with HTLV-I are common in southern Japan, the Caribbean, and some parts of Africa. In late 1987 a Red Cross study found that 10 units of American blood out of 39,898—or 1 out of 4,000—were infected with the virus.[35] Based on these figures it was estimated that 2,800 transfusion recipients a year would become infected with HTLV-I through the blood supply in the United States. According to the Red Cross's own calculations, this would make HTLV-I a greater transfusion risk than the AIDS virus.

In December of 1988, more than a year after these results were reported, and half a year after the Presidential AIDS Committee strongly urged such action, the FDA finally approved a test kit for HTLV-I. Like the AIDS test, the HTLV-I test detects antibodies to the virus rather than the virus itself. Consequently, like the AIDS test, a major problem with HTLV-I testing is that no one knows how long a "window period" exists between infection and the development of detectable antibodies. It should be remembered that the HTLV-I

*A retrovirus is a special category of virus whose genetic material is coded differently from other viruses so that it can be incorporated into an infected cell.

virus, like the AIDS virus, is a retrovirus and that it may take months or even years from the time one becomes infected and capable of passing the disease on to others until detectable antibodies show up in the blood. During this time, the infected individual is capable of passing the virus on because he or she will test normal despite the presence of infectious virus in the blood.

In the United States, HTLV-I has been most prevalent in the rural South. Recently, however, rising infection rates have been reported in large cities like New York, Miami, and Atlanta. Among intravenous drug users in New York, HTLV-I prevalence was 9 percent.[36]

HUMAN T-CELL LEUKEMIA VIRUS-II

Human T-cell leukemia virus-II(HTLV-II) is a retrovirus closely related to HTLV-I. It was discovered by Dr. Robert C. Gallo and Dr. David Golde in 1982. Like HTLV-I, and like the AIDS virus, HTLV-II is thought to be spread through blood, sexual intercourse, and shared needles.

Although there is not enough data yet, some researchers believe that HTLV-II can cause "hairy cell" leukemia, a rare but lethal disease in which the virus was first isolated. In the laboratory, the virus converts normal white blood cells to leukemic cells. However, its origins remain mysterious and there are concerns that it may cause other serious diseases. Until recently, retroviruses like HTLV-I, HTLV-II, and the AIDS virus were not known to cause infections in human beings at all. In animals, retroviruses have long been known to cause cancer.

HTLV-II was thought to be extremely rare until it began showing up among intravenous drug users in the United States in the period 1988–89. Various studies—in New Orleans, New York, San Francisco, and Los Angeles—have showed the virus to be present in anywhere from 5 to 20 percent of drug addicts, an alarming development that has baffled experts.[37] A survey of blood donors in San Francisco found HTLV-II to be more widespread than the AIDS virus. Another puzzling aspect of the virus is its appearance among groups not known to be at high risk for infection.

The new test that screens blood for HTLV-I is also believed to identify HTLV-II. The two viruses are so similar that the test cannot distinguish between them. No cases of transfusion-associated leukemia from HTLV-II have been reported to date, but this may be attributable to a long period of latency or the possibility that HTLV-II plays an indirect role in other cancers or lack of recognition of the disease.

SYPHILIS

After five straight years of decline, the number of syphilis cases in the United States is on the rise, in keeping with the overall surge in sexually transmitted diseases. Since 1985, cases of syphilis have increased by 30 percent to more than 86,000 annual new infections in 1988. The number is expected to rise again in 1990. The effects of full-blown syphilis are horrific: the disease can damage the heart, the nervous system, and the brain; it can also cause stillbirth or other birth defects.

The majority of new cases have been reported from Florida, New York, and California, but the numbers are up all across the country. Young women and heterosexual men, particularly inner city black and Hispanic populations, have been hardest hit by this increase, though all groups of sexually active men and women have been affected.

The blood supply has long been considered safe from syphilis because refrigeration of blood is supposed to kill the spirochetes (slender, spiral-shaped bacteria) that transmit infection. As a result, the AABB has proposed discontinuing routine syphilis testing for blood and blood products. However, given the growing number of syphilis cases, both in the United States and around the world, many medical experts now feel that syphilis testing should be mandatory.[38] Professor Ross Eckert, a member of the FDA Blood Products Advisory Board, argued the case persuasively in testimony before the Presidential Committee on AIDS in 1988:

The syphilis spirochete is killed by normal blood bank refrigeration, so blood bankers think the test is redundant. To see why this is wrong, play a mental game. Assume that you must be transfused and that you must choose between two bags of blood: one with dead syphilis spirochetes in it and the other without them. You would probably take the bag without the spirochetes on the common-sense presumption that any donor exposed to syphilis probably was sexually promiscuous and, if so, was more likely to have been exposed to other diseases that are neither detected by tests nor killed by normal refrigeration.

Until medical technology provides specific tests, "surrogate" tests like the syphilis marker are necessary to make blood safer.[39]

The increasing demand for fresh blood components, especially platelets, fresh frozen plasma, and blood for exchange transfusion in newborn infants, has also added to the risk of transmitting syphilis. Donors with latent syphilis can theoretically transmit the disease, and even after antibodies first appear, spirochetes can still be present in the blood.

MALARIA

Malaria is probably the most widespread disease in the world, with more cases of infection than any other. In some countries, the entire population is infected. Travelers returning to the United States from areas endemic with malaria are asked not to donate blood for six months. Infected individuals are barred from donating for three years.

However, since there is no practical, inexpensive lab test for malaria, American blood bankers must rely on a personal interview with prospective donors. As with AIDS, self-deferral is not a foolproof system. (In Europe, by contrast, self-exclusion is combined with testing for the malaria parasite.) Consequently there are still cases of malaria transmitted through blood transfusions in the United States, though they are not frequent.[40] Recipients who are chronically transfused and immunosuppressed patients are at the highest risk for infection with malaria.

Red cells are the most common and dangerous site for the malaria parasite. It can live in stored blood for up to two weeks though it is most infectious within the first 5 days. Since refrigerated blood must be used within 35 to 42 days, there is a good theoretical possibility of transmission. Frozen blood is not capable of transmitting malaria.

OTHER RARE INFECTIOUS BLOOD-BORNE DISEASES

Human immunodeficiency virus 2 (HIV-2) is a retrovirus in the same family as AIDS, HTLV-I, and HTLV-II. It is believed to be transmitted in the same manner—via sexual contact and blood—and it causes immunologic devastation similar to AIDS. Most cases of HIV-2 have appeared in western Africa—in some areas as many as 25 percent of those infected with HIV have HIV-2—with some cases in Europe and Brazil. While the disease is considered extremely rare in the United States, a 1989 study of several hundred specially selected blood samples in New York showed four confirmed infections of HIV-2 and two probable cases.[41] This represents the largest group of HIV-2 infection uncovered on this continent to date. Researchers are concerned that the full extent of HIV-2 remains unknown because there is no specific test to detect it. The standard blood test for AIDS antibodies to HIV-1 is the same test used to screen for HIV-2. Studies presented at the international AIDS conference in Montreal showed that between 45 and 90 percent of blood specimens with HIV-2 caused some reaction on HIV-1 tests. However, most experts concede that there is no way to gauge the number of HIV-2 cases that are slipping undetected into the blood supply.[42] Given our experience with HIV-1, and the fact that the first confirmed case of HIV-2 in the United States was reported only in 1988, further studies and tests are urgently needed, particularly in view of the high incidence of HIV-2 in some parts of Africa. Since HIV-2 is not being routinely checked, there may be a significant spread of this disease before the medical community becomes fully aware of its presence.

Chagas' disease is one of the most widespread diseases in the world after malaria, with over 12 million people infected in Latin America alone, from Argentina to Mexico. The disease is usually transmitted by a beetlelike insect known as the "barber beetle" because it bites sleeping victims in the face. The insect sucks out the blood and defecates on the wound, causing infection. In Brazil alone, there are a quarter of a million new cases of Chagas' disease from blood transfusions each year. The disease has yet to make serious inroads into the United States blood supply, although two American patients in the last three years were infected with Chagas' disease after blood transfusions. One of them died. Experts are concerned that other cases are going undetected because U.S. physicians are unfamiliar with the disease and do not understand that it can be spread via transfusions.[43] There are approximately 2 million people from Central and South America now living in the United States and about 100,000 of them are believed to be chronically infected with Chagas' disease. Immigration from these countries is also on the rise, making the potential for the spread of this disease through transfusions a growing possibility.[44] As of today, there is no effective treatment for Chagas' disease. In parts of South America, blood for transfusion is routinely treated to prevent the spread of Chagas' disease from a transfusion.

Serum parvovirus-like virus (SPLV), or B-19 virus affects children with sickle cell anemia and other patients with various forms of anemia. It has been known to cause arthritis, purpura, and spontaneous abortion. Between 25 and 30 percent of blood donors have antibodies to this virus. It can be transmitted through transfusion of blood and particularly through blood products like Factor VIII concentrate.

Brucella abortus, a bacteria, can survive in stored blood for several months and has been transmitted through transfusion. It causes fever, headache, chills, and muscle pains, and occasionally more serious complications like purpura and encephalitis. However, since it is normally present in donor blood at low levels, only patients with compromised immunity are generally at risk.

Salmonella septicaemia is usually transmitted through platelet concentrates and can prove fatal. One paid platelet-pheresis donor is known to have infected seven patients with septicaemia.[45] Between 1980 and 1983, the FDA recorded nine deaths due to posttransfusion septicaemia; of these, six were traced to infected platelet concentrates.

Toxoplasma gondii persists chiefly in white blood cells and so poses a danger mainly to immunosuppressed patients who are transfused with leukocyte concentrates. In the United States between 20 and 80 percent of blood donors have antibodies to this parasite, and about 18 percent may be actively infected.

Babesia microti, a parasite normally carried by ticks, can survive in stored blood for more than two weeks. It is usually mild with no symptoms but can prove fatal to splenectomized or immunosuppressed patients. One form of effective treatment has been exchange transfusion—the removal of the patient's blood and replacement with new blood. Babesia microti has only been reported in the northeastern coast of the United States, in Wisconsin, and Minnesota.

IMMUNOLOGIC REACTIONS

The most serious form of noninfectious complication resulting from a blood transfusion is a hemolytic reaction in which the transfused red cells are attacked and destroyed by the transfusion recipient's immune system. There are two basic causes for this occurrence. One is incompatibility of major blood types, which is usually due to human clerical error: a person with type A blood may receive type B blood by mistake. In such cases, the antibodies in the plasma of the type A recipient will interact with the antigens in the donor's type B red cells. All the type B red cells will be destroyed in the type A recipient, with extensive clotting and destruction of blood in the bloodstream. This type of reaction is usually immediate, and often fatal.

Fortunately, this kind of mixup is a rare occurrence. Between 1976 and 1985 the FDA reported 140 deaths as a result of mismatched donor blood (while cautioning that there was a serious underreporting of such fatalities). About half of those deaths were caused by errors at the bedside, meaning that the wrong blood was accidentally administered. Five people died because they received blood intended for their roommates.[46]

Another 25 percent of the 140 fatalities reported by the FDA were due to errors in the blood bank. These can include improper disinfectant and puncturing; an incorrectly administered test for compatibility and cross-matching; mislabeling or misplacing of serum samples; and too-long storage at room temperature. Inadvertent overheating or freezing of blood can also cause fatalities.

Although a small transfusion of incompatible red cells may lead to a severe hemolytic reaction, there is usually a direct correlation between the amount of blood transfused and the severity of the reaction. The higher the volume of transfused blood, the greater the risk. Hemolytic reactions usually occur very rapidly, within the first 15 to 30 minutes of transfusion.

While major incompatibility such as transfusion of type B blood to a type A person is rare, it is far more common to have minor hemolytic reactions due to undetectable antibodies in the recipient. Such reactions occur in about 1 out of 50 transfusion patients.[47] They are usually relatively mild, though severe reactions can occur.

Blood recipients who have had previous transfusions or pregnancies may have developed a special sensitivity or immunity to specific red blood cell antigens. The antibodies formed in response to these antigens, however, may not be detectable under routine compatibility tests. As a result, when transfusion is made with red cells carrying this specific antigen, the recipient's antibodies are stimulated in response. They attack the red cells as if they were an invading virus. A delayed hemolytic reaction occurs.

The antibody levels rise gradually over a period of days (7 to 10) until they destroy the transfused cells. Such reactions are not usually as severe as immediate ones. However, they normally involve a drop in the hematocrit,* which means that blood cells are being destroyed within the patient's body. Even delayed reactions many days after the initial transfusion may result in fever and chills, back pain, anxiety, jaundice, and general discomfort.

Moderately severe reactions can also occur as a result of heightened sensitivity to white blood cell and platelet antigens from previous transfusions or pregnancies. Symptoms include shaking chills followed by fever with anxiety and discomfort. Sometimes, acute respiratory distress and even pulmonary edema can occur. This is rare, but it can be fatal.

Plasma proteins with specific antigens may also produce allergic transfusion reactions accompanied by wheezing and respiratory distress. In rare instances, anaphylactic reactions occur, where the blood vessel walls collapse and one bleeds into the lungs. Citrate toxicity is another potential danger in transfusion reactions. Excess citrate from the anticoagulant preservative solution used in the blood collection bag occasionally causes a severe reaction in patients receiving multiple transfusions.

There is also the ever-present danger of bacterial contamination of blood and blood products. While these are uncommon with improved donor drawing and prompt refrigeration, bacterial contamination can lead to toxic shock syndrome: symptoms include nausea, severe shaking chills, vomiting, diarrhea, and shock, which can be fatal. All stored components of liquid blood must be regularly examined for any sign of bacterial multiplication such as gas bubbles, hemolysis, or turbidity. Frozen blood, by contrast, does not have this problem because blood is usually frozen shortly after collection and viruses and bacteria cannot multiply in frozen blood.

In some cases, circulatory overload may also produce a reaction. Many years ago, giving too much blood was a genuine risk, but today it is rarely encountered. The overriding problem now is lack of adequate transfusion. One out of every 100 transfusion recipients will experience a fever or rash as a result of accepting foreign blood into his or her system. And one in 100,000 recipients, or 30 times a year according to the FDA, someone dies from a mixup that leads to an attack on the red cells.[48]

Immunologic reactions are one way the body has of signalling us

*The hematocrit measures the percentage of red cells in the blood. See Chapter 7.

that it has been invaded by an alien substance. The culprit in such cases is not a virus or infectious organism per se, but an invader that can have a similar effect on the body's equilibrium: namely, human blood foreign to the recipient. Confronted by the entry of this intruder, the body's natural immune system may seek to counterattack, creating a potentially severe and even fatal chain of events.

As will be clearly shown in Chapter 8, "The Blood Bank of the Future," most of the risks enumerated in this chapter can be markedly reduced.

6

AIDS: A Special Case

The Human Immunodeficiency Virus (HIV)* epidemic will be a
challenging factor in American life for years to come and should be a
concern to all Americans. Recent estimates suggest that almost
500,000 Americans will have died or progressed to the later stages of
the disease by 1992. Even this incredible number, however, does not
reflect the current gravity of the problem. One to 1.5 million
Americans are believed to be infected with the human
immunodeficiency virus but are not yet ill enough to realize it . . .

Informed consent for transfusion of blood or its components
should include an explanation of the risks involved with the
transfusion of blood and its components, including the possibility of
HIV infection and information about alternatives to homologous
blood transfusion therapy.

*Executive summary and recommendation from the Presidential Commission on
the HIV Epidemic, June 24, 1988*

In the space of less than a decade an unknown disease has appeared
that has been variously described as nothing to worry about by
some authorities and the greatest threat to mankind by others. Not a
day goes by without a news report or TV story about some aspect of
AIDS. Often the information that the public receives is totally contra-
dictory. Most Americans are confused, fearful, and not surprisingly,
mistrustful of what they've been publicly told.

---

*Throughout this chapter, it is important to keep in mind that HIV is simply another
term for the AIDS virus.

AIDS is an elusive disease. Like the virus that transmits it, AIDS continues to elude detection and full comprehension. There are still basic, unanswered questions concerning the nature of the disease, its origins, and all the routes of transmission. The more we find out, the more troublesome seem the conflicting claims of so-called AIDS experts.

However, there are some undeniable facts about AIDS that we do know for certain.

AIDS is a relatively new disease. The first reported cases of AIDS in the United States were in New York and California in June 1981.[1] It is important to remember that diseases such as smallpox, syphilis, and leprosy have been recognized for hundreds, even thousands of years. The data on AIDS is still coming in.

AIDS kills. It is a fatal disease that has claimed human lives in over 100 countries. Death usually occurs between eight to ten years after the onset of infection, though it can occur in one to two years as well.

AIDS is infectious. It is caused by a virus and spread primarily through sexual contact, blood, and the sharing of contaminated needles. It may also be passed through the bloodstream from mother to infant and even from nursing infant to mother.

AIDS is insidious. The AIDS virus may live in the human body for years before noticeable symptoms appear. Most people who have AIDS are unaware they are infected.

AIDS does not discriminate on account of sex, race, or age. Anyone can get AIDS.

In Africa and some other parts of the world, AIDS is a heterosexual disease, affecting men and women equally. In the United States, AIDS was originally termed a homosexual disease, because it seemed to affect gay men disproportionately. Later intravenous drug users replaced gay men as the fastest-growing group of AIDS-infected patients in the United States. In 1990 heterosexuals appear to be the fastest-growing group of new AIDS cases.

As of today, there is no cure and no vaccine for AIDS.

Given these sobering facts, AIDS has been officially called the number one public health problem in America. Yet, despite this acknowledgement, the government and the scientific establishment have failed to inform and protect the public adequately. Where so much uncertainty exists, supreme caution and unceasing vigilance would seem to be the best policy. Yet where AIDS is concerned, caution has often been thrown to the winds and full disclosure frequently sacrificed to other considerations.

For example, the public is constantly assured that the AIDS virus is fragile and "hard to get."[2] But according to experiments reported in the *Journal of the American Medical Association,* the AIDS virus is quite hardy and can live on a dry surface for 3 days and on a wet surface for 15 days at room temperature.[3] Although these experiments were conducted on above-average concentrations of the AIDS virus, such potential durability hardly suggests a weak or frail organism.

The AIDS virus has also been isolated from saliva, although no instance of mouth-to-mouth transmission has yet been reported. However, in January 1989 the *Journal of the American Medical Association* published original research by a team of Italian physicians that documented mechanisms by which AIDS-infected blood cells could be transmitted by kissing.[4]

These doctors studied 45 healthy heterosexual couples and found that the amount of blood in saliva, normally present in 50 percent of subjects, increased significantly after toothbrushing and after passionate kissing. The presence of blood in saliva indicates microlesions or small tears in the oral mucosa, the special tissue lining the inside of the mouth. During kissing, these tissues, which can easily be torn, come into close contact and blood can pass directly from one subject to another. Passionate kissing increases the chances of passage through these small tears in the mouth. As a result, if the blood of one partner is infective, he or she can pass the HIV virus into the bloodstream of the other partner. The Italian team of doctors concluded with a warning that "passionate kissing cannot be considered safe sex for the transmission of human immunodeficiency virus infection."[5]

Human saliva has also been successfully used as a test medium for the detection of AIDS antibodies. In April 1989, scientists from the Roche Institute and St. Luke's–Roosevelt Hospital reported in the *New England Journal of Medicine* that they were able to detect 70 percent of AIDS-contaminated samples when using saliva from AIDS-infected subjects.[6] The scientists recommended developing a simple saliva test as a standard for AIDS virus detection instead of the present blood test.

There have also been documented cases of laboratory workers who were infected with HIV as a result of accidental spills. While these cases involved higher concentrations of HIV than usual, they strongly suggest that the AIDS virus is tougher and more resistant than commonly believed. To date, the Centers for Disease Control has reported 19 cases of American health workers who were accidentally infected with the AIDS virus. But according to David Bell, chief of the CDC's AIDS activity and hospital infection program, the figures are seriously understated: "We now know they're notoriously underreported. Basically, nobody knows how many health care workers have been infected on the job."[7]

Three large studies have placed the risk of contracting the virus at about 1 in 250 if a health care worker is accidentally stuck with a contaminated needle. Nationwide, accidental needle sticks occur more than 2,000 times a day, according to one study. Since the proportion of patients with HIV infection has increased in recent years, the CDC's count of accidentally infected health care workers should have increased more than it has, according to some experts.[8]

Although the CDC and other hospitals have been reluctant to admit this knowledge publicly, their recommendations for dealing with AIDS-contaminated material are totally consistent with the view that AIDS is a very hardy and dangerous virus. That is why extensive decontamination procedures are used in AIDS hospital rooms, including the wearing of secure protective garments. If the virus were so fragile that mere exposure to air for several minutes would incapacitate it, these stringent procedures would be unnecessary.

Estimates about the number of Americans infected with HIV have diverged widely. However, most of the estimates have been steadily, sometimes subtly, rising. The conservative figure, established by the U.S. Public Health Service in 1986 and supported by the Presidential Commission on AIDS, is that between 1 to 1.5 million Americans are currently infected with the AIDS virus.[9] Of these, about 30,000 were originally thought to be heterosexuals who had no other risk factors, according to the CDC. Other government estimates have recently been revised upwards and place the number of nondrug using heterosexuals infected with HIV somewhere between 80,000 and 165,000.[10]

Dr. William H. Masters, Virginia E. Johnson, and Dr. Robert Kolodney, in their controversial 1988 book, *Crisis: Heterosexual Behavior in the Age of AIDS,* argued that these figures were true two to three years ago, but were now badly outdated. They contended that the AIDS epidemic, like any sexually transmitted disease, was spreading rapidly because there was as yet no known cure or vaccine.

Most people who are infected with HIV do not know they have the virus—a point made by the Presidential Commission as well—and these infected subjects have been continuing to transmit the disease to a widening circle of contacts. Using these calculations, Masters, Johnson, and Kolodney estimated that the original 1.5 million Americans infected with the AIDS virus had now become 3 million infected carriers.[11]

However, the most controversial suggestion by the authors of *Crisis* was that of these 3 million carriers, about 200,000 were heterosexuals with no other risk factors—or seven times the CDC estimates at that time.[12] (The CDC estimates have since been revised upwards.) Masters, Johnson, and Kolodney argued that AIDS had long "broken out" of its original high risk groups and was now running rampant in the heterosexual community.

While *Crisis* was quickly dismissed for its lack of experimental rigor, a few months later the Hudson Institute, a private nonprofit research organization, estimated that the number of Americans infected with HIV was more than twice the government's estimate, somewhere between 1.9 and 3 million as of the end of 1987.[13] Even more dramatically, the Hudson Institute researchers, using a sophisticated computer model, suggested that infection among heterosexuals was three times as high as the government's latest, revised estimate, placing the figure between 200,000 and 500,000.[14]

Any serious estimate of the risks of contracting AIDS from a blood transfusion must be based on the prevalence of this disease in the general population. Unfortunately, this has been, and continues to be, a sensitive, controversial subject,* especially since many groups oppose the idea of nationwide AIDS testing, which is the only sure way to gather hard data about the disease. But even the most conservative estimates about the number of HIV-infected Americans today—between 1 and 1.5 million—indicate that this disease poses a far greater transfusion risk than is commonly acknowledged.

THE BODY'S NORMAL DEFENSE MECHANISM

To understand the risk of contracting acquired immune deficiency syndrome, it helps to understand how the body normally copes with disease. The human body is constantly attacked by all sorts of potential invaders. These invaders may be as large as insects or other parasites which can be seen with the naked eye. Some merely bite

---

*This is true for worldwide figures as well. In November 1989, the World Health Organization estimated that there were 6 million to 8 million people infected with AIDS worldwide, and that this number was expected to double or triple in the 1990s.[15]

through the skin to obtain blood while others try to burrow into the human body itself.

Of far greater significance are the much smaller invaders, called bacteria, that are only visible under a microscope. Bacteria multiply within the body but outside of the cells. In some instances, they can also invade the cells.

Even smaller than bacteria are supersmall organisms called viruses. While bacteria can be seen under a regular microscope, it takes the magnifying power of an electron microscope—capable of magnifying 50,000 times—to expose a virus to human sight. Viruses are so minuscule that they must usually invade the cells of the body in order to live and multiply. They are like alien life forms that attack and take over control of the cell, forcing the host into submission and reproducing themselves from within the host cells.

The human body has developed elaborate mechanisms to deal with these invaders. The first line of defense is our external armor, or skin. Most bacteria and viruses cannot penetrate through an intact, healthy skin.

The internal parts of our body are protected by a second mode of defense, a tissue known as mucous membranes. All the internal cavities of our bodies—mouth, stomach, intestines, nose, anus—are covered by these membranes. This internal skin is far more vulnerable to invasion by foreign microbes than our outside skin, because certain secretions and substances can pass relatively easily through these membranes.

The model of the common cold, and of how the body fights off this virus, is useful for understanding what does and does not happen during AIDS.

The air we breathe is filled with thousands of living organisms that move constantly in and out of our lungs as we take in life-sustaining oxygen and expel the waste gas carbon dioxide. As a result of this exposure, we are far more vulnerable to upper respiratory infections than to other kinds. The common cold, for example, is really a group of symptoms in which the membranes in the nose and throat are attacked and infected by viruses—viruses that usually progress no further. If an infection develops beyond the upper respiratory tract to the lungs, it is called pneumonia.

The frequency of pneumonia compared to the common cold is very low because in most healthy individuals the invading organisms get no farther than the nose or throat. With some, the organism does not even establish a beachhead at this upper site. These individuals seem to have a higher degree of natural resistance and may remain healthy when everyone around them is ill.

Once the cells in the throat are attacked by a cold virus, it takes the body only a few days to realize it has been invaded by a foreign organism. Immediately, specialized cells called lymphocytes begin to make antibodies against this assault. These antibodies are specifically shaped to tackle the invading virus, fitting it like a lock and key. We might also say that the antibodies form a "lasso" that collars the foreign invader.

Once the antibody attaches to the virus, special cells called leukocytes, or white cells, are able to grab the invader, swallowing and destroying it. Without the presence of antibodies to lasso and halt the invading virus, the white cells would be unable to capture it. (This description is somewhat picturesque and simplified, but enables one to visualize what is happening at a microscopic, biochemical level.)

After an infection is brought under control, the antibodies diminish in the blood—but some always remain. Once a viral invader stimulates the creation of antibodies, it is very difficult for that virus ever to establish a beachhead within the body again. As soon as the virus tries to reenter the body, preexisting antibodies will neutralize and destroy that virus before it has a chance to reproduce.

When an unprotected person is exposed to measles, for example, that virus quickly spreads beyond the mouth and throat and invades the whole body. A severe rash results. Within five to seven days, however, the body produces millions of antibodies and the mopping-up operation against the virus begins.

If the same person is exposed to the measles virus years later, there will always be enough measles antibody to quickly put the virus out of commission.* A healthy person would not even know he had been exposed to another episode of measles because the body would attack the virus and destroy it within hours.

However, there are situations in which a body is not capable of completely destroying an invading virus. Sometimes a virus may lie dormant within the body until certain environmental factors reduce

---

*If that is the case, many people ask, then why does one continue to get colds? The answers is that cold symptoms are caused by hundreds of different viruses. A healthy person does not catch a cold from the same virus twice. For this reason, children have many more colds than adults. By the time we reach adulthood, we have experienced many more viruses and formed protective antibodies that children do not yet possess.

the system's immunity or resistance: then it begins to multiply and cause symptoms. Fatigue and stress are well-known causes of a decrease in generalized immunity. Sometimes the onset of one viral illness can cause another illness that has been hidden to erupt. One example is cold sores or fever blisters commonly seen in the mouth.

Cold sores are due to a virus called herpes 1 or 2. This virus is latent in one-half of the U.S. population. A person is only infectious or capable of transmitting the virus when he has an open blister or sore. The sore indicates that the virus has become activated as a result of lowered resistance or immunity. Anyone who has ever had a cold sore is harboring some of these viral organisms, hidden in cells around the mouth, lips, and gums. Genital herpes, seen on the penis or in the vaginal region, is another variety of the herpes virus. It is unpleasant but rarely life-threatening. As in the mouth, infection occurs only when blisters or sores are present.

It should be clear that the model of the common cold or the measles—where, within a few short days, the body makes an antibody that permanently wipes out the virus—does not hold in all situations. This brings us to AIDS.

THE AIDS VIRUS

AIDS (acquired immune deficiency syndrome) is caused by a virus now called HIV or human immunodeficiency virus. HTLV-III, or human T lymphotropic virus III, is sometimes also used. AIDS is the final stage of infection with the HIV virus. By the time a person has the symptoms of AIDS, his immune system is so damaged that he is susceptible to a variety of infections that are normally harmless to a healthy person. A special form of cancer, called Kaposi's sarcoma, can also occur because of the breakdown of the immune system. AIDS is, strictly speaking, not a single disease but a syndrome or collection of different diseases that attack and exploit the body in the weakened state created by the AIDS virus.

In addition to being almost incurable, the AIDS virus has some very special characteristics that make it difficult to detect. In contrast to most viral infections, where the body forms effective antibodies in five to ten days, with AIDS this process is normally delayed for an indefinite period. Previously it was believed that most AIDS-infected people formed antibodies in 6 to 14 weeks. Recent studies suggest that it may take three years or more for antibodies to be produced.[16]

There are other rare cases in which no specific AIDS antibodies are ever produced.[17]

This deadly delay occurs because the AIDS virus has the special ability to invade the T-4 lymphocytes,* the very cells that make antibodies. The long gap between the invasion by HIV and the recognition by the body that it has been invaded suggests a sinister science fiction plot in which aliens surreptitiously invade the body and force the host to reproduce more aliens, multiplying and taking over the body in a manner too subtle to detect until it is too late.

The AIDS virus attacks the T-cells, penetrating through the cell wall and moving into the nucleus, the control chamber of the cell. Once inside, the virus releases a strand of genetic material that takes over control of the host's genetic material, forming a fatal, indissoluble bond.

The invaded cell, instead of reproducing itself, now produces more alien invaders, ensuring the destruction of the host. Infection is permanent, since the virus is now integrated into the genetic code.

After it has infiltrated the nucleus, the virus lies dormant and waits for the signal that will activate it. Many studies now suggest that the AIDS virus becomes active and multiplies when the body is responding to new challenges such as other diseases. Herpes, hepatitis B, and syphilis have been known to trigger this response.

When the biochemical signal arrives for the T-cell to start replicating and activating the rest of the immune system, the AIDS virus steps in and instead reproduces itself, killing the host cell and eventually the body. The very system designed to defend and protect an individual from outside invasion becomes the agent of his destruction from within. In order for the disease to spread as it is currently doing, however, that individual has to infect others and continue the process of immune sabotage.

In addition to the T-4 lymphocytes, the AIDS virus also attacks and impairs other cells that are part of the immune system: B cells, monocytes, and macrophages.

Macrophages are special white cells that not only travel in the bloodstream but can move into various organs like the brain. Once these cells are colonized by the AIDS virus, they become vehicles for transmitting the disease instead of combating it. The brain is a com-

*T-4 lymphocytes are white blood cells critical in the body's immune response. The T-4 cell count is a measure of the state of the immune system based on the number of T-4 lymphocytes present in the blood.

mon target for such transmission. Sometimes the first sign of AIDS infection is mental confusion, known as dementia.

Another chilling element of AIDS is its long, clandestine incubation within the body. According to most authorities, including the Institutes of Medicine, the average length of time between infection and diagnosis is "at least eight years."[18] An individual infected with HIV may not suspect that anything is wrong for many years. During this interval, he may infect countless other people who will also be contagious but similarly unaware that they have the disease. They in turn will spread the disease to yet other unsuspecting individuals.

Most cases of AIDS are not detected until an individual becomes visibly sick and is then tested. The overwhelming majority of the 1.5 to 3 million Americans now infected with AIDS do not yet know they have the disease. Of the 500,000 Americans expected to die or reach the later stage of AIDS by 1992, only a few more than 100,000 cases had been reported by the CDC as of October 1989. Of these, more than half, or about 65,000, had died.

If these estimates by the Presidential Commission and others are correct, then about 400,000 Americans will develop full-blown AIDS in the next three years. This amounts to 130,000 new AIDS victims and about 75,000 new AIDS deaths each year.* Today we are still not prepared—medically, economically, socially, or psychologically—to deal with the threatened deluge.

For the same reason, people who received blood transfusions between 1977 and 1985—before the AIDS-antibody test—are still considered at risk for the disease.[19] The first recommendation of the Presidential Commission on AIDS was to mandate "look-back" notification and inform recipients of blood or blood products since 1977 of their possible exposure to HIV.[20] The commission also recommended that blood banks voluntarily test all transfusion recipients since 1977 for possible exposure to AIDS. So far blood banking organizations have not responded to this request. Even if they do comply, it will take at least until 1993 for the full tally of prescreening transfusion-AIDS cases to be measured. Of even greater importance is the one obvious step that no one has yet recommended: that every person who receives a blood transfusion today should have a follow-up blood test within one year to ensure that they do not inadvertently

---

*Due to serious underreporting of AIDS cases, the real number of infected persons, and of AIDS deaths, is no doubt much higher already, making the expected additional deaths correspondingly lower.

spread the disease to their partner, and to enable them to seek improved treatment for their own infected state. Given what we know today about the long window period between infection and the appearance of AIDS antibodies, a follow-up blood test at six-month intervals *for several years* is advisable.

AIDS AND SOCIETY

The epidemic of AIDS, which is now only in its early stages, is destined to change the order of American society and probably the world as well. One of few positive changes that might result from this scourge is the ultimate restructuring of the blood banking system to a much safer form than now exists.

The lag time between the discovery of a danger and an appropriate public response is sometimes incredibly long. There was at least a 15-year period during which evidence accumulated that asbestos was toxic and caused cancer before it was outlawed as an insulating material. The cost to society of removing asbestos years later is many times greater than it would have been had appropriate measures been taken early on.

Similarly, the danger of radiation causing cancer and other injury to the body was known for at least 15 to 20 years before strong measures were taken to limit exposure. We shudder today when we consider the unnecessary radiation that American volunteers were exposed to in the early years of atomic testing. Yet even before the atomic era, there was evidence that radiation was dangerous and life-threatening.

Historians will look back in amazement at the opportunities that were missed to contain the transmission of AIDS before it spread to millions of people in the United States. At the present time there are an estimated 1.5 to 3 million infected people who continue to spread AIDS through society without adequate safeguards. In high-risk urban areas like New York, AIDS is still not classified as a communicable or sexually transmitted disease. In 1987, the New York State Society of Obstetricians and Gynecologists sued the State Health Department to change this classification, but they lost the case in court. While there are serious civil rights issues involved, such considerations must be weighed against public health concerns. Laws applying to syphilis or gonorrhea, which were specifically passed to protect society against the spread of these sexually transmitted diseases, are not enforced against the politically sensitive AIDS. More significant, with new drugs, improved treatment, and greater knowledge about AIDS, early detection may enable HIV-infected persons to live longer, healthier lives once they are identified.

We may be deluding ourselves in an effort to avoid unpleasant choices, trading off present discomfort for future upheaval. Eventually this disease may destroy many of the freedoms we now take for granted. The scope of the ultimate damage will depend on how long we delay instituting basic public health measures to contain the spread of AIDS.

AIDS AND THE BLOOD SUPPLY

Ever since the introduction of HIV testing in March 1985, official estimates of the risk of contracting AIDS from a blood transfusion have ranged from 1 in 250,000 to 1 in 100,000.[21] Blood banking organizations (such as the American Red Cross and the AABB) and federal agencies (such as the FDA) have consistently assured the public that the nation's blood supply is "virtually safe" from transfusion-AIDS.[22] The CDC, which has been, relatively speaking, a little more vigilant and more forthcoming than other organizations, has acknowledged that the risk of AIDS in transfusion might be as high as 1 in 40,000 units. But the American Red Cross has disputed these CDC figures, claiming in a 1989 *New England Journal of Medicine* article that the chances of becoming infected with the AIDS virus through a blood transfusion may be "fourfold fewer than reported previously."[23] The Red Cross placed the estimate at 1 infected unit per 153,000 units of blood transfused, or almost four times lower than the official CDC estimate.

However, these figures are all somewhat misleading. To begin with, the risk estimates are based on the risk per transfusion component, not per person. Remember that whole blood is commonly broken down into several components such as red cells, plasma, and platelets, each of which is transfused separately. According to the American Red Cross's own calculations, the average transfusion involves 5.4 units of blood.[24] In other words, the average transfusion recipient is exposed to 5.4 units of blood—red cells, platelets and plasma—or more than five times the risk represented by the 1 in 153,000 figure. A more direct way to state the Red Cross risk estimate would be to say that each blood recipient faces a 1 in 28,000 risk of contracting AIDS through a blood transfusion.

However, even this 1 in 28,000 figure seems highly optimistic. By comparison, the CDC estimate, when divided by the average 5.4 unit transfusion, translates into a 1 in 7,400 risk of contracting AIDS for every transfusion recipient. While 1 in 7400 is not a high risk, neither is it negligible, especially when one recalls that 4 million Americans each year are exposed to blood transfusions. When one considers that the incidence of transfusion-AIDS in high-risk urban areas like New York is believed to be five to ten times higher than in the rest of the country,[25] these numbers take on new significance: a risk of 1 in 740 to 1 in 1,500 for every person receiving a blood transfusion in New York is considerably higher than public estimates indicate and suggests that a much more cautious approach to blood transfusions may be warranted.

Despite the fourfold lower, and more recent, Red Cross figures published in the October 5, 1989, *New England Journal of Medicine,* the CDC has stuck by its original estimates. Dr. John W. Ward of the CDC pointed out that the American Red Cross does not collect blood in New York City, large parts of Texas, and San Francisco, thus omitting some of the highest risk AIDS areas from their findings and possibly skewing the results.[26]

Another serious flaw in the 1989 Red Cross study was that the authors used an average window period—the time between infection with the AIDS virus and the appearance of AIDS antibodies—of 8 weeks. The researchers acknowledged that estimates of transfusion-AIDS risk are "very sensitive to the length of the window period" and that if the eight-week period were extended even to ten weeks, their risk analysis would increase by 25 percent.[27]

Yet even a ten-week average window period may appear like wishful thinking. An increasing number of studies, including one presented at the international AIDS conference in Stockholm in 1988, have shown that AIDS antibodies may not form for over a year.[28] On June 1, 1989, a major new University of California study was published by the *New England Journal of Medicine* showing that AIDS antibodies may not form for three years or more.[29]

While there is still much controversy and debate surrounding the exact length of the window period, it seems reckless to assume a best-case scenario of eight weeks when much longer window periods have been clearly documented—and when human lives are clearly at stake. The American Red Cross researchers acknowledged that the

chief risk of HIV infection in the blood supply was due to the indefinite window period, but then they went on to disregard evidence that
showed a widening gap between the time a blood donor is infected
with HIV and the time the donor's blood begins to test positive on
current antibody tests.[30]

Even the CDC can be faulted for some aspects of its AIDS-tracking
role. For example, CDC estimates of the incidence of transfusion-
AIDS are compromised by the fact that they do not include people
who may have contracted HIV from a blood transfusion but died
from their operation before they could develop AIDS. This group
constitutes a sizeable number since the CDC itself estimates that 50
percent of the people who receive a transfusion die. CDC officials
have admitted that they are only "guessing" about the risks of HIV
transmission through the blood supply and that their figures are
rough estimates, since there are no direct measures of the number of
AIDS-infected units of blood that escape detection.[31] It is important
to keep these qualifications in mind when discussing the potential
risk of contracting AIDS from a blood transfusion.

The CDC is open to other criticisms. In 1988, it was cited by the
Presidential Commission on AIDS for its "lack of strong leadership in
the public health community for obtaining and coordinating HIV
infection data."[32] One of the biggest problems is that the CDC does
not keep track of people infected with HIV, but only those who have
full-blown AIDS. Since it takes, on average, ten years before HIV
infection turns into clinical AIDS,* this means tht the CDC figures
are rather low and may represent only a small fraction of the infected
population.

While AIDS survival rates have improved with new drugs and better care, medical experts across the country now concede that almost
all individuals who are HIV positive have AIDS, even if they appear
healthy because they are still at an earlier stage of the disease.[33] There
has been a great deal of public confusion about the distinction between HIV infection and AIDS. HIV infection simply means that one
has AIDS with no symptoms. If you have HIV, you are infected with
the AIDS virus. Restricting the term to those who have symptoms is
tantamount to saying that if you have cancer with no symptoms, you
don't have cancer.

---

*For those infected with AIDS through a blood transfusion, the average period
between infection and the appearance of clinical AIDS symptoms is seven years.

Official reassurances concerning the low risk of contracting AIDS from a blood transfusion belong in a league with statements by tobacco companies claiming there is no, or hardly any, link between cigarette smoking and cancer. Anyone with the slightest appreciation of medical statistics knows that smoking not only causes lung cancer but lip cancer, mouth cancer, and heart disease and emphysema as well. Yet it took a surgeon general's report and years of legal activism to get the message out that cigarettes kill people and damage the infants of mothers who smoke.

Blood transfusions carry a profoundly higher risk of transmitting AIDS than is being acknowledged by most blood banks. The sooner these risks are admitted, the easier it will be to protect the population from unnecessary infection. The quantity of blood needed to transmit HIV infection is incredibly small. Studies in the December 1989 issue of the *New England Journal of Medicine* have shown that a single pint of AIDS-contaminated blood contains enough virus to infect 1.8 million people.[33a]

To understand the real risk of transfusion AIDS one needs to know the occurrence of detectable AIDS in the blood supply *after* so-called high-risk individuals have been screened out. According to present guidelines, all male homosexuals, bisexuals, intravenous drug users, and prostitutes and their associates are supposed to be eliminated in a prescreening process in which a medical history is obtained. Blood will not be taken from any individual with these risk factors.

There do appear to be some unsettling exceptions. In May 1988 in New York, a homosexual newspaper called *Gay Scene* was charged with running advertisements for blood donation. The ads were created by the Greater New York Blood Program, a joint venture between the New York Blood Center and the American Red Cross aimed at soliciting blood donors. The New York Blood Center, however, denied that they had sent the ad.[34]

A spokesman at *The Advocate,* another gay publication that is sold nationally, was quoted as saying that his paper did not run public service announcements, but that he thought it was all right for homosexuals to donate blood.[35] In San Francisco, gay newspapers continue to run blood recruitment ads and have threatened to sue for discrimination if the ads are pulled. In the predominantly gay and lesbian Castro neighborhood in San Francisco, gay leaders successfully lobbied against efforts to withdraw community-based blood drives. After intense pressure, in August 1988, Irwin Memorial Blood Bank voted to reinstate the blood drives in the Castro.[36]

Despite many precautions, the prescreening process, which asks high-risk donors to exclude themselves, is not working adequately. Self-deferral is not, in itself, an adequate protection for the blood supply. Despite improved education, high-risk persons are still donating blood today. Some feel socially pressured not to reveal their sexual preferences; many are unaware they are infected, or erroneously think they do not belong to a high-risk group: for example, some men who are predominantly heterosexual but occasionally have sex with men do not consider themselves homosexual; others donate blood as a means to get an anonymous AIDS test; and a few individuals have knowingly donated infected blood. Meanwhile, several recent studies in both the *Journal of the American Medical Association* and the *New England Journal of Medicine* have shown that the majority of people who donate infected blood still belong to high-risk groups, despite the much-publicized campaigns for self-exclusion.[37]

There is also the danger of human error in handling blood.* In 1985, the FDA admitted that 13 units of HIV-contaminated blood had been released for transfusion through error. According to an article in *Science* magazine, 10 of 19 laboratories that applied to conduct AIDS-antibody testing for the Army had error rates of 5 percent on at least one occasion.[38]

In March 1988, the American Red Cross recalled 24 units of contaminated blood that had been released to hospitals in Washington, D.C. and Nashville, Tenn.[39] Two senior officials of the Washington regional Red Cross Office were suspended for 30 days pending an investigation. The FDA, responding to criticism of its own close relationship with the Red Cross, agreed to step up inspection of Red Cross collection centers to once a year instead of once every two years.

In July of 1988 the FDA cited the Red Cross for 152 violations of procedures in dealing with blood during the preceding year and a half. The procedures dealt with the screening of blood for the viruses that cause hepatitis B and AIDS.[40]

In September, following new inspections, the Red Cross announced that 2,420 contaminated units had been mistakenly released, most of them from four regional centers. A month later the Red Cross announced a voluntary recall of 1,400 units of blood that were improperly tested for AIDS over a three-year period in Los Angeles. Most of the blood and blood products had already been used

---

*Even in an autologous system, there is always the danger of error, but there is additional protection. See Chapter 8.

and obviously could not be recalled.[41] These findings of human error and testing mishaps are all the more troubling because there is no retesting of blood initially found to be HIV-negative.

Any blood sample deemed antibody-negative by an HIV screening test, the ELISA test, is automatically approved for transfusion, without any backup procedure. No second test is conducted. As soon as the blood sample gets a preliminary clearance, it is judged suitable and safe for use. However, the present HIV screening test is known to have a false negative rate of at least 2 percent.[42] This means that out of every 100 samples of infected donor blood screened, the test may erroneously report that 2 are free of antibodies when antibodies are actually present. These two units of blood, infected with HIV, will then be approved for transfusion. The ELISA test for AIDS antibodies may prove even less accurate when AIDS infection is in its earlier, lower-antibody stages. Some studies have found an ELISA false negative rate for AIDS antibodies as high as 5.8 percent.[43]

False negatives occur when the antibody is present just below the limit of detectability. Unfortunately, this blood is highly contagious when used for a transfusion. But even without this margin of error in the ELISA test, we now know that the AIDS virus may not cause the formation of antibodies in some people for several years. These individuals would appear healthy and test negative for HIV, yet they are capable of transmitting infection when their blood is used for transfusion. Another group of individuals known to be infected with AIDS have been shown to lose their antibodies after several years.[44] An indeterminate number may never develop antibodies at all.[45]

In fact, a much bigger problem than false negatives—people who have AIDS antibodies that are missed by the test—is the problem of people who are infected with the AIDS virus but *have no antibodies*. Even if the ELISA antibody test was a perfect test and picked up everyone with antibodies, all those people who have the AIDS virus but no antibodies would still be missed. Just as the first line of defense, donor self-deferral, has proved inadequate, so the second line—an AIDS antibody test performed on every sample of blood—has been shown to have major flaws.

According to a July 1989 study in the *Journal of the American Medical Association,* 1 out of 5,000 blood plasma donors infected with the AIDS virus was found to be negative by the standard AIDS antibody test. The blood of these undetectable AIDS-infected donors slipped past the screening test and was accepted into the general blood supply because of the "window" period.[46]

The most ominous finding appeared in a major study published in the *New England Journal of Medicine,* June 1, 1989,* which found that HIV infection may occur at least 35 months before antibodies to HIV can be detected.[48] According to this study, which to date has not been disputed—though it has been largely ignored or misrepresented—[49] *infection with the AIDS virus may remain undetected for three years or more despite the use of the standard AIDS-antibody test.*

In this study, conducted by researchers at the University of California, 133 healthy homosexual men who initially tested negative for AIDS despite persistent involvement in high-risk sexual activity were followed for several years. Researchers used a special test, too difficult to perform in standard laboratories, which can detect the AIDS virus itself, unlike the standard test, which can detect only AIDS antibodies.

Of the 133 men, 31 became infected with AIDS and were followed for three years after proven infection. All 31 AIDS-infected men remained outwardly healthy during this time. Astonishingly, only 4 out of the 31 infected men tested positive on the standard AIDS antibody test within a 36-month period.[†]

In other words, 87 percent of the infected but healthy-appearing men were undetectable by the standard AIDS screening test after three years of infection. These men were slipping through a very wide "window." In effect, for every AIDS carrier detected within the three-year period, there were seven undetectable carriers.

Previous studies had suggested that most individuals become positive for AIDS within three months of infection. If you did not test positive within six months, you were generally considered free of AIDS. Now it seems that these figures may be seriously in doubt.

Earlier studies showing the development of AIDS antibodies in three months or less seem to be based on cases of people who developed acute symptoms resembling those of mononucleosis, often accompanied by a rash, shortly after exposure to a known AIDS carrier.

---

*The *New England Journal of Medicine* study came one year after a Northwestern University School of Medicine study by Dr. Steven M. Wolinsky, which found that of 18 homosexual men, 14 were infected for more than a year before developing antibodies. After the June 1, 1989, study confirmed these ominous findings, one of the researchers was quoted by the *New York Times* as saying that "several other well-respected laboratories would soon publish similar results" but that "everybody was trying to proceed in as responsible and conservative a way as possible."[47]

†Of these four, not one showed up positive for the first ten months.

Within about two weeks of the onset of this illness, patients began to feel better and developed the asymptomatic HIV carrier state. People with this kind of picture almost always went on to develop AIDS antibodies within 3 months. However, it now seems possible that in a significant number of AIDS-infected individuals there is no outward sign of infection and, even more ominously, there is no development of AIDS antibodies that can be readily detected.

The authors of the *New England Journal of Medicine* report cautioned that the degree of infectiousness in these delayed-antibody patients was unknown.[50] While these healthy, high-risk homosexual patients may have lower quantities of the AIDS virus in their blood than those who show antibodies after three months, they clearly have enough virus to cause infection. One should keep in mind that AIDS infection can be contracted from a needle prick in which only a single drop of AIDS-contaminated blood is involved. By contrast, a person receiving a single transfusion of blood would be exposed to the equivalent of 5,000 to 10,000 drops of blood (one unit of blood equals about 500 milliliters; one milliliter contains from 10 to 20 drops; remember that one pint of HIV-contaminated blood can potentially infect 1.8 million people).

Of particular significance in the June 1, 1989, study was the fact that all the infected men had virus cultured and grown from small samples of their blood.[51] This was incontestable proof that these men harbored live, active AIDS virus capable of reproducing. A transfusion from any one of these men would contain more than 100 times more blood than the blood sample that was used to grow out the live AIDS virus, and so would be particularly likely to transmit AIDS infection to anyone who received blood from such an individual.

These findings obviously have very serious implications for the safety of the blood supply. They suggest that individuals harboring the AIDS virus within their blood may remain outwardly healthy for years, yet nevertheless be capable of passing AIDS on to other individuals via blood transfusions. If the "window" period for the appearance of AIDS antibodies may be at least three years, then the current AIDS-antibody or ELISA test is of limited use for blood donors. It also raises very serious questions about the adequacy of testing for AIDS carriers in the wider population.

These problems occur because the present ELISA test is an indirect marker for the disease, not a direct test. It only measures AIDS virus antibodies, not the virus itself. As a result, infected individuals continue to slip through. In a letter published in the *New England Journal of Medicine* in August 1988, almost a year before the University of California study, Dr. Alan Salzberg, chief of medical service at the Veteran's Administration Medical Center in Miles City, Mont., estimated with his associates that up to 7 percent of people carrying the AIDS virus are in this "window of infectivity" period.[52] (Other studies have put the figure at 6 percent.)[53]

Based on their calculations—Salzberg and his associates used a computer model—the Veterans Administration medical chief and his fellow researchers claimed that as many as one in every 5,000 people who undergo major surgery in the United States may become infected with AIDS-tainted blood.[54] In high-risk areas like New York, Salzberg and his associates estimated that the risks might be ten times as high, infecting one in every 500 people who received a transfusion.*

Of course the number of people potentially infected far exceeds the number of contaminated donations that slip through. This occurs because each blood donation is broken up into an average of three components—red cells, platelets, and plasma. And each component can itself carry HIV infection. Therefore, each infected donor may transmit AIDS to at least three separate people from one donation.

The danger is greater because, as discussed earlier, the average transfusion recipient gets 5.4 components of blood. These five or six components are never from the same donor, since it requires too much time and effort to keep them together. Each component, however, is individually capable of transmitting the AIDS virus. Therefore a patient who receives an average 5.4 unit transfusion might easily be exposed to five or six potentially infectious donors. A patient who receives *two* transfusions might actually be exposed to 11 donors. The danger of contracting AIDS for such a patient living in New York cannot be ignored.

While New York State has the highest percentage of AIDS cases in the United States, the risk of AIDS from a blood transfusion is not confined to the Northeast. In fact, through 1986, New York had 33 percent of all AIDS cases nationwide, yet only 18 percent of all transfusion-associated AIDS cases.[55] Conversely, 34 percent of transfusion-AIDS cases came from states with fewer than 23 percent of all AIDS cases. These figures seem to suggest that transfusion-AIDS is,

*The estimate made by Salzberg et al. was based on an average of 8-unit transfusion for major surgery, which is higher than our 5.4 average. On the other hand, new studies have shown that their 1.5-month average "window" period is too low.

relatively speaking, even more of a threat in rural communities previously thought to be at low AIDS risk.

A 1988 review of a Midwestern blood bank revealed that 989 out of 659,439 donors, or .15 percent tested over a two-year period, were positive for the AIDS virus.[56] This would be about 1 in 650, which is three times higher than the .05 percent or 1 in 2,000 figure reported by New York State between October 1985 and March 1988.[57]

In May 1989, the *New England Journal of Medicine* published a joint study from Houston and Baltimore claiming that risk of contracting AIDS through the blood supply was low.[58] The figure quoted by the Houston-Baltimore study was .003 percent, which translates into 1 in 33,000. However, once again, the figure referred to the risk per transfusion component, not per person. In this study, the average patient received 11 blood components, so that the risk *per patient* was actually about 1 in 3,000, a far more worrisome figure.

The official CDC estimate of contracting AIDS from a blood transfusion—1 in 7,400 nationwide, possibly five to ten times higher in cities like New York—stands as a conservative but sobering warning. The original estimates made by Dr. Salzberg and his associates were even higher—1 in 5,000 nationwide, 1 in 500 in New York—though they have since been substantially reduced.[59] Masters, Johnson, and Kolodney, using a third method—based on new HIV cases who slip through the window period, and previously infected people who test falsely negative—came up with a strikingly similar figure of 1 in 5,418.[60] However, their figures were based on the risks of becoming infected via transfusion from a single component of blood, as opposed to a single transfusion. Since the average transfusion involves at least five components, the Masters, Johnson, and Kolodney figure would average out to 1 in 1,000. The Houston-Baltimore study, despite claiming that the risk of transfusion-AIDS was low, reveals on closer examination a not-insignificant 1 in 3,000 risk per patient.

It is clear that several independent medical researchers, using dissimilar analytic methods, have produced similar conclusions; while no one knows exactly how high it is, the risk of HIV infection from a blood transfusion in the United States is far higher than generally acknowledged. The Houston-Baltimore study alone should give pause for thought, not least because of the misleading reassurances it draws from its own data. If the risk of acquiring AIDS to the average blood recipient is 1 in 3,000 in medium-risk areas, one must consider the consequences for transfusion recipients in cities like New York and San Francisco.

All of the above figures, however, could become obsolete by the startling finding that a significant number of healthy AIDS carriers do not appear to develop detectable antibodies for at least three years. It is now painfully clear that the risk of contracting AIDS from blood transfusions is nothing like the 1 in 153,000 figure officially cited by the American Red Cross—even if we "translate" the Red Cross figure into a 1 in 28,000 risk per patient. A far higher number of individuals, in some areas possibly 1 in 750 or even higher, are currently being exposed to AIDS when they receive a blood transfusion. It is important to recall that 50 percent of the entire hemophiliac population in the United States became infected with the AIDS virus at a time when the blood banking establishment was reassuring the public that there was nothing to worry about. At the present time, this tragedy may be in the process of being repeated, but on a far greater scale.

THE DEADLY DOUBLE STANDARD

Understandably enough, both the government and the medical establishment have downplayed the risks of transfusion-AIDS. Yet among themselves, public health authorities and many professional blood bankers understand the real dangers only too well. Perhaps the most telling proof is the fact that there are two classes of blood transfusion recipients in the United States.

In February of 1988, the CDC, without revealing all its information, suddenly recommended that sperm used for artificial insemination in the United States be frozen and stored in quarantine for six months.[61] First, a blood sample taken at the time of sperm donation was to be tested and found free of HIV antibodies. Then, a minimum of six months later, a second blood sample was to be taken from the same sperm donor and tested again to make sure no antibodies had developed over the six-month period. Since it was erroneously believed that almost all people infected with AIDS develop antibodies within six months, the sperm of a donor who still tested negative after this interval could be released for use.

According to the CDC and the FDA, who collaborated on the report, even if the sperm initially tested negative for the AIDS virus, it was not to be used, since there was a long latent period before sufficient antibodies might develop to be detectable. Retesting the donor after six months provided a safety net and an opportunity to double-check the original diagnosis. Only by freezing and storing the semen and by retesting the donor's blood six months later could one with reasonable certainty eliminate a very significant number of AIDS carriers who showed up negative on the first test but who were actually infected. (While there was still the danger of antibodies that would not show up for several years, a six-month quarantine was a good first step that would catch a significant number of AIDS-infected individuals that might otherwise slip through.)

One of the most striking aspects of this formal recommendation issued by the government—and immediately accepted as the new "standard of practice"—was that it applied *only* to sperm. Blood could be used immediately without retesting the donor six months later for any signs of HIV infection.

While sperm donors and blood donors undergo identical AIDS-antibody screening tests, one crucial difference is that a blood transfusion is known to be at least 1,000 times more infectious than sperm. The CDC has shown that a single transfusion of AIDS-contaminated blood carries at least a 95 percent chance of infection.[62] In other words, whereas it may take multiple exposures to the sperm of an HIV-infected partner before one becomes infected with AIDS, a single transfusion of AIDS-infected blood will almost certainly lead to AIDS infection. With blood, there is no second chance.

If, as the FDA and CDC were openly admitting, an AIDS test at the time of the initial sperm donation was an inadequate guarantee of sperm safety, then what about blood? Why was blood safe with only a single AIDS test at the time of initial donation while sperm was not? Why weren't similar precautions being taken to protect blood recipients from the AIDS virus?

It is both inconsistent and irresponsible to claim that sperm must be stored in frozen quarantine for months and not used until the donors are retested because of the significant risk of AIDS, while at the same time claiming that there is no significant risk from blood transfusion, when blood is known to be so much more infectious than sperm. Yet today there is still no quarantine period for blood. Donated blood is used immediately after one initial screening, with no safety precaution for the dangerous window period.

Not only is blood much more infectious than sperm, but blood also affects the lives of far more Americans each year. According to the U.S. Government Office of Technology Assessment, there are approximately 172,000 women who undergo artificial insemination each year, while there are 4 million recipients of blood transfusions annually. Obviously the risk of AIDS infection is far greater for the general population. Why weren't 4 million transfusion recipients being protected with the same safeguards that apply to those who receive artificial insemination?

In a private meeting with FDA officials in the summer of 1988 I inquired how it was possible to issue such a regulation for sperm while permitting blood to be used without a storage and quarantine period. No satisfactory answer was given, although concern was expressed about potential shortages in the blood supply system. However, the answer to the real feelings of the FDA about the safety of the blood supply came out in a little-publicized memorandum sent out by the FDA to plasma collectors in October 1988.

The private FDA memorandum, published by the American Blood Resources Association in the November 1988 issue of *Plasmapheresis*— a technical magazine for the industry—called on all blood recipients involved in special antibody collection programs to receive only frozen blood, stored for six months, from donors who were originally tested for AIDS and hepatitis, and then retested six months later. The recommendations for a changeover were clear and unambiguous. "The donors of the immunizing red blood cells should test negative for all referenced infectious disease markers both at the time of their initial donation and at least 6 months later on a freshly drawn sample."[63]

This was, coincidentally, the same program we advocated and pioneered when we opened the first autologous blood bank in the United States in 1985. The concept of freezing blood and retesting donors three and six months later, which was then—and still is—resisted by most segments of the blood banking establishment, had overnight become official policy in a private communication to a limited segment of the plasma-collection industry. However, almost all members of the medical profession, most members of the blood-banking establishment, and the public at large were completely unaware of the creation of this select group of blood transfusion recipients.

In its present form, this new guideline is highly selective and discriminatory. It creates a double standard in which members of the general public are deemed to be less important than a select group of paid donors. These special plasma donors are to receive their minitransfusions only from blood donors who have been tested after a six-month interval to guard against infection with HIV and hepatitis—an open acknowledgment that the present testing system is inadequate. However, no one else is to be protected with these same safeguards.

Who are these special blood plasma donors who are paid to produce selective antibodies and are now receiving such special treatment?

In the United States, there are limited numbers of individuals willing to receive tiny transfusions of blood incompatible with, or not matching, their own. These individuals, who receive less than 1/20 of a normal transfusion, subsequently have a small transfusion reaction which produces antibodies. This antibody-rich blood is collected at a later time, and the plasma portion is then used to make special blood-testing reagents and injectable products.

Such individuals, referred to as "source plasma donors who consent to receive selective immunization," are paid for taking these risks. In order to protect them against HIV and hepatitis infection, the red cells they receive are now to be tested and frozen for six months, while the blood donors who provided those red cells are themselves retested six months later to make sure they are still free of infection. Only then can the quarantined blood be released for use.

The real question now is how long the public will tolerate a system that needlessly exposes it to infection with the AIDS virus. A single donor slipping through the system is likely to infect three recipients, since blood is separated into at least three components. Each of these infected individuals will then more than likely cause secondary AIDS infections. A single infected donor may thus cause the transmission of AIDS to three to six people from one donation—and even more in a nonmonogamous situation.

There is increasing documentation—and I have seen several such cases myself—of people who have contracted AIDS from a blood transfusion and proceeded, unwittingly, to infect their spouses.[64] In a much-publicized case, a Marine officer sued the federal government, alleging that Navy doctors gave his wife an AIDS-tainted blood transfusion that eventually killed her, killed their son, and is slowly killing him.[65] The case of Chief Warrant Officer Martin Gaffney has not yet been decided by the courts, but it points to the potential for multiple tragedies resulting from a single transfusion of contaminated blood.

In another well-publicized case, TV star Paul Michael Glaser, formerly of "Starsky & Hutch," lost his seven-year-old daughter to AIDS as a result of a blood transfusion that his wife received.[66] Mrs. Glaser contracted the AIDS virus from contaminated blood and unwittingly passed it on to her daughter through breast-feeding. Her five-year-old son was infected in the womb but has not shown any symptoms yet. Three members of one family have thus been infected from a blood transfusion, and one has already died. The full extent of such secondary and tertiary infection is seriously underestimated.

The number of infants infected with AIDS from blood transfusions is also disproportionately high. In fact, the first case of blood-borne AIDS occurred in an 18-month-old-infant who was repeatedly transfused. It is not generally appreciated that infants sometimes require multiple small transfusions. Although they make up only 2 percent of all transfusion recipients, infants account for more than 10 percent of transfusion-AIDS cases. As of December 1988, the CDC reported that 13 percent of children infected with AIDS were believed to have acquired the virus through blood transfusion, and 6 percent from blood products used to treat hemophilia.[67] This means that one fifth of children infected with AIDS in the United States have contracted the disease as a result of unsafe blood.

While such preventable tragedies unfold, unjustifiably low figures are still cited and false claims made for the safety of the blood supply. The same week in which a new study revealed that AIDS antibodies could be latent—and hence undetectable—for over a year, the American Red Cross reiterated its misleading assurance that the chance of acquiring AIDS from a blood transfusion was 1 in 250,000.[68] By the time the *New England Journal of Medicine* reported that AIDS antibodies might not show up for more than three years, Dr. Lewellys F. Barker, senior vice president for blood services of the American Red Cross, responded to these findings by assuring the public that the blood supply was "as safe as we can make it."[69]

If AIDS can be undetectable for as long as three years or more by current laboratory tests, then at any given moment a significant number of apparently healthy people are walking around in an AIDS-infected state of which they are unaware. These people may donate AIDS-contaminated blood, which will slip undetected into the blood supply. While no one knows the exact number of AIDS-infected units in the blood supply, the risk of contracting AIDS through a blood transfusion is significantly higher than the public has been led to believe. If we are to make a mistake, let us err on the side of caution and grant maximum protection to all blood recipients rather than repeating the tragic mistakes made prior to 1985 that caused over 20,000 Americans to be transfused with AIDS-infected blood.

Until a specific, practical test is devised that can directly detect the presence of the HIV virus, and so eliminate the window period, blood transfusions will not be safe from AIDS. As of today, there is no such test—yet one needs urgently to be developed. It should be the number one priority of the FDA and of organizations like the American Red Cross and the American Association of Blood Banks which are entrusted with protecting the nation's blood supply. Until such a test becomes widely available and affordable, the blood supply will not be, in the words of the current claim, "as safe as we can make it."

7

Undertransfusion

Blood transfusions once were believed to be relatively safe, but many physicians and patients recently have come to regard them as potentially dangerous. . . . The number of homologous blood transfusions should be kept to a minimum.

National Institutes of Health, "Consensus Conference," Journal of the American Medical Association *260, no. 18 (1988)*

In 1986 Donald Manes, a New York politician under formal investigation, attempted suicide by slashing his wrists. Manes was rushed to a hospital where, according to newspaper reports, his physicians elected not to give him a blood transfusion because of the fear of AIDS and hepatitis.[1] One can assume that his physicians felt that although he had lost significant amounts of blood, Manes was still at a sufficient level not to require a transfusion. Instead, they replaced Manes's lost blood with sterile salt water.

Approximately 36 hours after his initial bleeding episode, Manes experienced crushing chest pains. He was rushed to the intensive care unit where he reportedly received four pints of blood. By this time, of course, it was too late to prevent his heart attack. He had simply lost too much blood, and his heart was starved of oxygen.

Manes apparently lost between one-third and one-half—or even more—of his total blood volume. An individual his size would have approximately ten pints of blood in his body. Since Manes received a transfusion of four pints, and since no one is fully replaced with blood, we can safely assume that Manes lost at least half of the blood in his body. Yet his doctors withheld a transfusion until it was too late.

It is important to emphasize that this case is not exceptional and that Manes's physicians were behaving in the generally accepted fashion. Yet the Manes case illustrates something rarely discussed in public: the withholding of blood from patients who have suffered extensive blood loss. As with Manes, blood is frequently replaced only after the development of disastrous consequences. Mr. Manes managed to survive his heart attack and leave us with a public record of a case that demonstrates the kinds of complications that may result from undertransfusing severely blood-depleted individuals.

The Manes case also underscores the difficulty of gauging blood loss accurately when the standard tests, the hemoglobin or hematocrit count, are used. These standard tests are simply an inadequate measurement of the amount of blood lost, particularly when bleeding occurs over a relatively short period of time, such as a few hours.* Manes's physicians apparently believed that Manes had been bleeding for only "ten minutes"[2] and, based on his initial blood tests, they greatly underestimated the amount of blood he had lost. Clearly, Manes's physicians did not realize that Manes had lost more than half the red cells in his body; otherwise they would not have waited until he had experienced a heart attack to transfuse him with four pints of blood. It is worth noting that all of Manes's blood loss was from a slashed wrist and that this bleeding was stopped as soon as he reached the hospital. We know therefore that all of Manes's blood loss occurred prior to his admission to the hospital, and yet his blood count tests at the time of admission after his bleeding had been stopped, and the tests a few hours afterward, failed to reflect the true extent of the massive bleeding that had taken place earlier.

Despite claims that people are being overtransfused with blood, I cannot recall seeing a single patient suffering from this practice within the past ten years. Yet I have personally seen patients who experienced strokes and heart attacks from being undertransfused; and occasionally I have also seen severely anemic patients with unexplained sudden deaths wherein the most likely culprit was undertransfusion.

The physician today is faced with a genuine dilemma in treating patients with blood loss: to try to balance the risks of transfusion with potentially infected blood against the risks of undertransfusing patients. In almost every case, the physician will choose to un-

---

*Surgery is a typical situation in which patients lose large amounts of blood over a short time span.

dertransfuse his patient, and in most cases his judgment as to the safe level of undertransfusion will prove adequate; his patient will survive despite being deliberately undertransfused. Unfortunately, as in the Manes case and in many other unreported cases, the physician may misjudge the extent of the blood loss and the degree to which a particular patient can tolerate the deprivation of blood until a catastrophe occurs. The Manes case offers the public a rare glimpse into the unacknowledged risk of undertransfusion because the details of his medical emergency were published in the newspapers. Similar details of private cases are protected by physician-patient confidentiality.

A major complication leading to such errors of undertransfusion is the difficulty of measuring actual blood loss. There is no single direct way of measuring the blood volume that an individual has. It can only be done through a difficult test that involves hours of measurement and calculations. Even then, the best estimate has an error rate of plus or minus 10 percent.*[3]

The standard practice is to perform a hematocrit or hemoglobin test, which actually measures blood thickness, not volume. The body's ability to thin out and redistribute the remaining blood is often impaired, and this process may take hours or even days, distorting the hematocrit reading. Therefore it is common to seriously underestimate the amount of blood lost because the hematocrit is artificially high. This occurs because the remaining blood in the body has not yet been fully diluted.

Several past studies have shown that the decrease in blood volume during an operation is greater than expected, judging from the amount of blood lost externally.[4] One experiment showed that less than half of the blood loss occurred during the operation. Another quarter of the blood was lost within the next 24 hours; and almost a third of the total blood loss took place in the week *following* the operation.[5] In other words, doctors are consistently underestimating the amount of blood lost by their patients and replacing even less of the blood than they think has been lost. A surgeon may believe that his patient only lost two pints of blood when he actually lost four pints. I have observed this in many of my own patients; their ultimate

---

*A recent development called the BVA 100, or Blood Volume Analyzer, currently under review by the FDA, will provide for the first time a way of measuring blood volume rapidly and accurately to within 2 percent. I was associated with the research and development for this instrument.

blood loss cannot be fully recognized until ten days after surgery. These patients are being undertransfused because the full extent of their blood loss goes unrecognized.

Simply put, undertransfusion means that patients are not getting the optimum amount of blood for their medical and surgical needs. As a result, their chances of recovering from trauma or from surgery may be seriously impaired. Strokes and heart attacks are complications of major surgery that can be caused by inadequate blood levels. These complications involve a significant number of patients each year and result in unnecessary deaths.

The true incidence of strokes and heart attacks resulting from undertransfusion is unknown, but it clearly exists. The Manes case is only one example of this problem, which merits serious attention and further research. In the past two years, two patients I treated suffered heart attacks as a result of undertransfusion*—serious medical events that might have been avoided. Clearly, if a blood transfusion were as safe as infusing sterile water, no physician would hesitate to transfuse a patient with blood.

To understand the nature of the problem, one must keep in mind that not only is the safest blood for transfusion your own, but the safest *amount* of blood to have when one is medically ill or facing surgery is a full, normal quantity of blood within one's body. This would seem self-evident. Yet there are many responsible doctors who maintain that it is really not necessary to have a normal amount of blood when one is facing an illness. Such views defy both common sense and experimental studies showing that the addition or subtraction of even one pint of blood makes a significant difference in a person's physiological functioning.[6]

As a result of the known risks of transfusion, independent hospital transfusion policies have been established that create significant new risks for the patient. All the current guidelines for transfusion are based on the desire to avoid giving blood except when absolutely

---

*Most hospitals have transfusion committees that will not permit individual physicians to order blood for replacement unless a certain level of loss has been reached. In the two heart attack victims I treated, the patients had significant blood loss, yet their hematocrit levels remained above the minimum 30 percent transfusion guideline, so that neither the hospital transfusion committee nor the surgeon felt that a blood transfusion was warranted. In many hospitals, a physician does not have the authority to order a transfusion for a patient who has bled significantly down yet remains above the minimal hematocrit level unless that patient has stored his own blood ahead of time.

necessary. Motivated in large part by fear of AIDS, both doctors and patients are permitting situations of severe blood loss to occur without replacement transfusion. In practice this has meant that blood is regularly withheld from patients who could benefit from its therapeutic use.

This withholding of blood for transfusion affects two kinds of patients. The first are those who suffer involuntary blood loss, such as trauma resulting from an accident or any one of dozens of medical conditions that may cause internal bleeding. Instead of replacing this lost blood, hospitals initially administer sterile salt water as a volume replacement. This has the effect of thinning out the remaining blood in the body. Only after enormous amounts of blood have been lost, usually 3 to 4 pints out of a total volume of 8 to 12 pints, does replacement with blood begin.

Today it is common practice to use salt water replacement in an 80-year-old man who has lost as much as three or more pints of blood. Since bleeding from any cause amounts to an "involuntary" donation of blood, an 80-year-old man who has lost three pints of blood is no different from one who has just donated three pints. Yet until the AIDS crisis and the new blood shortages it created, it was considered dangerous for anyone over the age of 65 to donate even one pint of blood.

Since there is no precise way to measure the amount of blood that a person has lost, and since doctors are increasingly reluctant to risk a transfusion, patients are now commonly permitted to lose massive quantities of blood, which are replaced only with sterile water.

A second form of undertransfusion is the current practice of donating one's own blood prior to surgery. This practice is based on the desire to avoid a transfusion with someone else's blood. While in itself a good idea, the type of "autologous donation" that is currently practiced has some significant risks that may outweigh its benefits.

In this form of autologous donation, patients donate up to five pints of their own blood in the weeks before their operation.[7] As a result, they frequently begin their surgery, and undergo most of the procedure, with significantly lower blood levels than normal.[8] Hence, just when they most need all their strength, they may be missing up to a third of their normal red blood cells. This lack of red blood cells—the carriers of oxygen—significantly hampers the patient's ability to withstand the operation and to recover postoperatively without added complications.

Many physicians feel that it is worth trading off the risk of operating on a patient with his own thinned-out blood for the benefit of reducing that patient's need for outside, potentially infected blood from the general supply. And, to the extent that a patient can make back his own blood in the days before surgery, this approach is sensible. However, most patients do not have adequate time to make back their own blood before surgery. As a result they start out with lower blood levels and need even more blood than someone who enters surgery with a full, normal volume—in addition to the blood autologous donors lose during the natural course of the operation, they also need to get back the blood they predonated. Consequently, they cannot be adequately restored to a normal blood level unless they receive additional outside blood—and thus defeat the whole purpose of their predonation.[9] The only other alternative is to undergo the operation in an anemic and blood-depleted state and to remain in such a state in the recuperative period—and this is, in effect, what frequently occurs.

The practice of undertransfusion is based on several common misperceptions. It is routinely claimed, for instance, that patients who are missing one, two, or even four pints of blood—more than a third of their total red blood cell volume—do not need a transfusion.[10] Yet the FDA has itself ruled that a donor may give blood only once every eight weeks. Under the best conditions, a young, healthy adult male may make up the loss of a pint of blood within twelve to fourteen days. Older individuals may require from three to five weeks to replenish their lost red cells, while elderly people may need as much as one to two months to make up the loss of a single pint of blood.

The FDA directive prohibiting healthy people from donating more than once every eight weeks makes good sense from a safety point of view. By contrast, the present guidelines for preelective autologous donation, initiated in 1984 in response to the AIDS scare, are seriously flawed and place patients at significant new risk in their effort to avoid a potentially infected transfusion.

In experiments reported in the July 1988 issue of the *Journal of the American Medical Association,* doctors followed AABB standards for autologous donation before elective surgery.[11] They found that after only the second unit of blood was removed in two weeks, one quarter of their patients were already anemic. Before the researchers were finished, 71 percent of their subjects became anemic simply from predonating their own blood. Rather than being aided and fortified, these patients were actually weakened prior to facing the rigors of an operation.

   The AABB guidelines for preelective autologous donation, theoretically permitting five or even more blood donations within a five-
week period, are therefore demonstrably unrealistic and even
counterproductive for patients facing surgery. As can be seen from
the study cited above, patients rarely get to donate more than one
pint or two before problems with anemia develop. The optimum
situation is to begin and end any operation with a normal supply of
blood. To the degree that a patient is operated on with a below-
normal supply of blood—or has to undergo the postoperative state
with less than a normal supply—that patient is exposed to additional
risks. Thus the only appropriate method for predonating blood is to
do so well in advance, in order that the body may have time to replace
what it has lost.

   The new regulations governing autologous blood donation were
passed in an effort to minimize the risks of transfusion and to compensate for the devastating loss of donors that hit the blood banking
industry when AIDS was first publicly linked to transfusion. Some
donors were prevented from giving blood because they belonged to
groups at high risk for AIDS. Many stopped donating because of the
erroneous impression that they could get AIDS from doing so. Some
experts estimate that the industry lost about one-third of its donors in
the immediate aftermath of the transfusion-AIDS connection.[12]

   Other rules governing blood banking were also changed in an
effort to restore and expand donor recruitment. The minimum age
for blood donors was reduced from 18 to 17 so that high schools
might furnish a potential new source of supply. Of even greater
significance, the maximum age for blood donors was raised from 65
to 75 years and upwards, depending on the discretion of the blood
bank physician.[13] For autologous donors, it was now stated, "there are
no age limits."[14]

   One asks whether there is any medical authority in the world who
would recommend that a *healthy* seventy-year-old should donate two,
three, or four pints of blood to someone else at any time. If the answer
is no (and it is), then how can an *ailing* seventy-year-old donate that
much blood when he himself is about to undergo surgery? In truth,
the last person who should give blood is a patient about to have an
operation where she will herself be losing blood. The loss of even a
single pint can decrease the patient's oxygen-carrying capacity below
a threshold level so that the additional stress of surgery combined
with anemia may cause disastrous consequences. It is often difficult to
know, particularly in the case of older patients, whether a person has

narrowed vessels in the heart or brain. Sometimes the first indication of such narrowing occurs when a blood-depleted person suffers a heart attack or stroke.

Recent studies have shown that removal of only a single pint of blood from a healthy athlete results in a measurable decrease in performance. Experiments conducted at San Diego State University showed that runners experienced a noticeable deterioration in their running times after donating one unit of blood.[15] It was not until four weeks later that the runners approached or equaled their original mark. If it thus takes between two and four weeks for a young, healthy athlete to return to previous levels of cardiovascular performance, a 70-year-old, like most older people, will be far slower in making up new blood. The loss of one pint, or more, can have serious conse-quences for such a patient about to undergo surgery.

An average person pumps the body's entire volume of blood through the circulatory system in one minute. At rest, an individual with ten pints of blood in all would pump those ten pints completely through the system in 60 seconds (at a heartbeat or pulse of 60, 1/6 of a pint is pumped per heartbeat). The pumped blood is distributed to all the key areas in the body, the most critical areas being the heart and brain. Blood supply to the brain must be steady and constant, and the heart, too, has to maintain an absolute baseline level of blood flow. These blood needs are continuous and vital.

Almost all the other parts of the body—limbs, intestines, liver, kidneys—can withstand a marked reduction in their blood supply if the needs of the body change. For instance, runners and swimmers who eat a large meal prior to competition may develop cramps and other difficulties. Athletic activity diverts blood away from the intes-tines to the muscles of the body. This diversion can be tolerated for limited periods of time, as long as it is only partial. A basic principle with respect to the blood supply, therefore, is that the system does not maintain a steady supply of blood to every part of the body at full flow all the time. Some areas are less critical than others and can make do with an irregular supply.

The body has an extensive control system that regulates the width of thousands of blood vessels throughout its network. The control of blood to various parts of the body is activated by minuscule, circular muscles that open or narrow the blood vessels like little gates; by widening or narrowing specific blood vessels, they can shift the blood preferentially from one area to another. When a weightlifter picks up a heavy weight, blood vessels open wide, increased blood flows through, and we see the arm and shoulder muscles bulging.

In a young, healthy individual, the blood vessels are smooth and clean, and these vessels contract or open wide depending on the needs of the body in that region. As a person ages, the vessels accumulate deposits of calcium and cholesterol. These deposits narrow the channels and make the vessels more stiff, so that they no longer open or close so readily. As these changes progress, the vessel openings grow narrower and narrower. In effect, a springy, rubberlike vessel becomes more like a little iron pipe with small rocky deposits inside. Blood flowing through such vessels is greatly slowed, even if the heart is pumping at a normal level. Often, even when the heart pumps harder, the amount of blood flowing through such vessels is only slightly increased.

This is a common occurrence is most human hearts and brains. As people get older, the majority develop this constriction of the vessels, called arteriosclerosis. If one is fortunate, these changes are mild and one retains relatively springy blood vessels that can respond to changing needs. However, in blood vessels where this constriction has occurred, the thickness of the blood is of critical importance in determining how much oxygen can get through to supply the body.

It is relatively common for individuals to have blood vessels that have narrowed by 75 percent or even 90 percent of their normal diameter through disease. Under these circumstances, the areas of the heart or brain that are supplied by these narrow vessels are severely compromised and at great risk. These compromised areas are very sensitive to blood loss or significant blood thinning, which may result in a critical drop in oxygen-carrying capacity.

Heart attacks commonly occur when a heart with a narrowed vessel attempts to pump more blood due to increased physical activity—and a blood vessel that has barely been able to supply enough oxygen under normal conditions can no longer deliver these additional requirements. Under these conditions, the heart muscle can be destroyed because it is deprived of adequate oxygen.

In essence, a heart attack is nothing more nor less than the destruction of a segment of the heart due to inadequate blood flow. It is only in recent years that cardiologists have begun to recognize that one does not need the complete closing of a blood vessel to kill a section of heart muscle. A mere falling of the oxygen level in the muscle below a critical point may cause a segment of heart muscle to die.

When one considers that individuals over fifty often have arteries narrowed by as much as 80 percent or more, and that the loss of even a single pint of blood decreases the oxygen-carrying capacity of an individual by 10 to 15 percent, one can better appreciate the profound risks of undertransfusion. To deprive the body of its regular supply of blood and to starve critical areas of adequate blood oxygen in the face of surgery is to invite disaster.

Normal human blood cells survive for only 120 days within the body. Individuals must therefore replenish their blood supply continually. A healthy person would ordinarily replace his entire blood supply three times in one year. Some individuals are chronically anemic—they have thin blood—because their ability to replace worn out red blood cells is limited. Even working at maximum capacity, the best an anemic person can do is sustain a red cell count at low normal levels, or levels slightly below normal. The practice of donating blood just prior to surgery almost invariably produces an anemic condition.

Strokes occur when a portion of the brain loses its blood supply. This can happen in several ways. A clot can form in a blood vessel, blocking supplies to that part of the brain; or the vessel can rupture, blocking further circulation to a portion of the brain. A stroke may also occur when a blood vessel narrows slowly so that there is less blood flow through the opening. Last, and most important, a stroke will take place if blood is so thinned out that it does not carry enough oxygen to the brain. A patient who has donated several pints of blood in the weeks prior to surgery may have a difficult time receiving adequate oxygen in those parts of the body where vessels are already narrowed. This is a common situation for people with arteriosclerosis, which results in narrowed blood vessels in the heart and brain.

The amount of oxygen carried by the blood is directly proportional to the number of red cells within the blood, as measured by the hematocrit. Hematocrit levels are crucial indicators in determining whether or not to transfuse a patient. The hematocrit measures the red cell mass, or the percentage of blood which is composed of red cells relative to the watery, plasma part. It thus reveals the thickness of the blood.

A normal hematocrit level for a man is 45 percent (see Table 1). This means that in a man, red cells normally make up 45 percent of the blood volume, with plasma or the liquid part of the blood accounting for the other 55 percent of blood volume.

A man who has a hematocrit of 24 has lost close to half of the red blood cells in his body. Some men, particularly the elderly, will not survive such blood loss. A man with a 30 hematocrit has already lost

Table 1 Hematocrit Levels: How Much Blood Are You Missing?

Hematocrit	Remaining Blood (%)
Men	
45	100
42	93
39	86
36	80
33	73
30	66
27	60
24	53
21	46
18	40
15	33
Women	
39–40	100
36	91
33	83
30	76
27	68
24	60
21	53
18	45
15	38

one third of the red blood cells in his body, or anywhere from three to four pints. Even a loss of one third of the body's red blood cell supply can result in serious complications, especially if the loss is rapid. It should be noted that blood loss is always greater than the hematocrit indicates immediately after an injury or illness, because blood does not thin out completely for several days. In humans, hematocrit levels below 20 are usually associated with major complications or death.

A normal hematocrit for a woman is 39 to 40 percent, which means that women have fewer red cells than men and more liquid plasma (about 60 percent). In women a hematocrit under 36 percent, and in men a level under 40 percent, is considered anemic. In effect, women start off with a lower red blood cell supply than men and, in situations of equal blood loss, they are more vulnerable than men.

A common transfusion guideline currently in use in many hospi-

tals is a hematocrit level of 30 percent. If the hematocrit does not
drop below this level, the patient will not be transfused. A 30 percent
hematocrit level for a man means that he is missing a third of the
oxygen-carrying red cells in his body (see Table 1).

At some hospitals, transfusion guidelines are even more severe.
After cardiac surgery, a patient with a hematocrit as low as 23 percent
might not be transfused. Under these circumstances, the heart has to
pump almost twice as much blood to deliver the same amount of
oxygen as it would with a normal hematocrit of 45 percent. Restoring
a patient's circulating red blood cell mass to normal levels before or
immediately after surgery would undoubtedly aid recovery and reduce the risk of a stroke or heart attack.

The hemoglobin count is another way of measuring blood thickness. Broadly speaking, each gram of hemoglobin equals three hematocrit points. Therefore a hemoglobin count of 15 would be roughly
equivalent to a hematocrit of 45 percent. A hemoglobin count of 10
and a hematocrit of 30 percent (known as "the 10/30 rule") is commonly used as a baseline for blood transfusions. If either the hemoglobin or hematocrit falls below this level, a transfusion is considered
advisable. In other words, fully one third of a patient's red blood cell
supply must be lost in order to merit a transfusion.[16]

Preoperative hemoglobin levels are considered an important determinant of postoperative mortality. A recent study in a New Jersey
medical center showed that patients whose hemoglobin levels were
below a threshhold figure were 16 times more likely to die than
patients with higher counts.[17] Of course, patients with lower hemoglobin levels, or more severe anemia, may well have more serious
illnesses and undergo more serious procedures that may have played
a role in their increased mortality. Nevertheless, these findings indicate that having a higher level of oxygen-rich blood significantly
increases a patient's chances for survival.

Blood loss during surgery is also a crucial determinant of mortality.
In the same study, patients who lost less than 500 milliliters of
blood—one pint is 650 milliliters—were five times more likely to
survive than patients who lost more than 2,000 milliliters. Put simply,
patients who lost less blood had a significantly better chance of survival.

Taken together, the two indicators make for very accurate predic-
tions of mortality. Out of the 125 patients tested (all of whom refused
transfusions for religious reasons), there were 17 deaths. However,
not one patient with a hemoglobin level above the threshold figure

and blood loss less than 500 mL died. The study, which appeared in the August 1988 issue of *The Lancet,* strongly suggests that adequate blood levels play a critical role, if not the most crucial role, in a patient's chances for surviving surgery. However, it should be pointed out that the authors of the *Lancet* study concluded that patients appear to require less preoperative transfusion than what is usually given, since the sharp increase in risk occurred at a lower hemoglobin concentration (eight instead of ten) than is usually used to indicate the need for a transfusion. This typifies the prevailing minimalist stance of asking what is the least one can get away with, rather than what is best for the patient.

Unfortunately, the *Lancet* study evaluated only whether the patient lived or died. It would have been useful also to tabulate the frequency of heart attacks and strokes related to blood levels in patients who survived. I have little doubt that such an analysis would show a higher incidence of strokes and heart attacks among severely undertransfused patients who lived.

The significance of adequate blood levels can also be seen in the dramatic results following treatment with erythropoietin in patients with end-stage kidney disease. In a recent, multicenter three-phase study reported by Dr. William Waters of Piedmont Hospital, Atlanta, treatment with recombinant human erythropoietin—a promising new drug that stimulates the bone marrow to produce red blood cells—rapidly and markedly improved the anemia in patients who were undergoing hemodialysis for end-stage kidney disease.[18] In addition to increased energy and activity levels and exercise capacity, marked improvements were seen in cognitive function, cardiovascular function, appetite, sex drive, and ability to sleep. Most significantly, many of the patients were able to return to work. According to Dr. Walters, "The administration of erythropoietin with elevation of hematocrit into the near normal range makes nearly as big a difference in the way the patients feel on a daily basis, as does the chronic uremic syndrome with dialysis."[19]

These findings further illustrate the critical role that adequate blood level plays in every patient's health condition and care. The minimal target that Dr. Waters and his associates used was a hematocrit level of 35 percent, after which the dose of erythropoietin could be reduced. This suggests that patients should have a higher minimal blood level than the standard transfusion guideline of 30 percent that is now recommended. The results of the study, which need to be followed up, give some indication of the vastly beneficial effects of human blood, presently undervalued and underutilized due to the current climate of fear and confusion. The study shows clear proof that blood-depleted individuals improve in every significant function that can be measured when their blood depletion is corrected. It should be noted that these patients were only partially corrected, and yet they showed dramatic improvement. One can only speculate about what additional degree of improvement they might experience if their blood depletion were corrected completely to normal.

A higher than 45 percent hematocrit—but no higher than 50 percent—seems to be an optimal level of blood thickness for athletic activities. As a result, some athletes resort to "bloodpacking" or "blood doping": they withdraw blood from their own bodies and train until their normal blood volume is restored.[20] Then, prior to competition, they retransfuse their own blood, gaining an extra unit of oxygen-rich blood and a higher hematocrit level. Athletes who prepare in this way have been shown to have supernormal capabilities, and the practice has been outlawed. In the 1987 world championships, skier Kerry Lynch was stripped of his silver medal when he admitted to blood doping.[21] In the 1988 Olympics, blood doping was apparently widespread, with several bicyclists admitting they had used the technique. But while the added advantage of one extra pint of blood may be unfair in formal competition, any patient facing a serious operation would want and is entitled to receive every possible advantage. And just as it makes little sense for an athlete to donate blood prior to a major athletic event, so is it medically unwise to remove blood from a patient about to undergo the stress of major surgery.

People who live at high altitudes naturally develop higher hematocrit levels as their bodies compensate for thinner oxygen. For years athletes have trained in high-altitude cities such as Denver to increase their blood counts and performance levels. Beyond a certain point, however, further increases in red cells do not effectively enhance the oxygen-carrying capacity of the blood. This may seem puzzling at first, but it is due to the fact that the amount of oxygen carried to an organ depends on how fast the blood is being supplied.

If the blood is too thick, or the hematocrit level too high, the thicker blood creates increased friction as it passes through the narrowed vessels. Under these circumstances, the advantages of extra oxygen in the blood are outweighted by the increased difficulty of pumping this thickened blood through the blood vessels. Up to a point, however, a higher red cell count or a higher hematocrit level is advantageous. An individual who has a hematocrit level of 20 percent has to pump blood at twice the rate of an individual wth a 40 percent hematocrit level to deliver the same amount of oxygen.

The rate at which blood is pumped in the body depends primarily on the heart muscle providing the pumping force. A 65-year-old whose blood has been thinned out to almost half-normal level must pump blood at twice the normal rate, 24 hours a day, just to supply the same amount of oxygen that could be delivered with half the effort if there were a normal red blood cell supply. Imagine the effect of this strain on the heart of an individual who during surgery has lost three or four pints of blood, which has been replaced with water.

BLOOD LOSS

Blood loss may result from hundreds of different kinds of medical problems. It can be slow or rapid. When the amount of blood lost rapidly is equivalent to 30 percent of total volume, a subject may pass into shock. Shock is a medical condition accompanied by extremely low blood pressure and inadequate blood flow to various areas of the body.

The sudden loss of as much as 40 percent of blood in the body will cause death in most cases, and the sudden loss of 50 percent of the blood supply will almost inevitably result in immediate death due either to stopping of the heart because of inadequate blood in the heart itself or to starvation of the brain. In traumatic accidents when an individual dies before help arrives, it is usually because of irreversible damage to either the heart or brain. Massive, rapid blood loss by itself may be the sole cause of death.

One of the humane ways of slaughtering an animal is to cut the jugular veins and arteries. Blood loss is so rapid that the animal is unconscious in less than 30 seconds and dead within minutes. An identical outcome occurs in human beings when blood loss is massive and uncontrolled. For this reason, a basic first aid rule is to compress the area of blood loss to prevent further bleeding.

In most blood loss situations treated in hospitals, individuals lose blood much more slowly. Even in traumatic accidents, victims are usually brought to a hospital where their blood loss is quickly stabilized and fluid replacement started. In those situations where blood loss is massive and rapid, with anywhere from one third to one half of a patient's blood lost in minutes, patients frequently expire before they reach the hospital. An individual can survive the loss of more than one half of the blood in his or her body, provided it occurs over a gradual period of time so that fluid within the body can enter the circulation. In many medical and surgical trauma situations, a small amount of blood may continue to be lost for a period of several hours. However, replacement is almost always initially by sterile salt water. It is very rare to give blood as the first replacement unless blood loss has been extreme.

Contrary to public perception, it is uncommon for a blood transfusion to be given in the case of injuries such as trauma resulting from a car accident. The overwhelming majority (over 88 percent) of transfusions are given for medical and surgical situations unrelated to accidents or injuries.[22] Patients with cancer, heart disease, and gastrointestinal disease are the leading recipients of blood transfusions, accounting for over 50 percent of transfusions each year.

"Exsanguination" is the medical term for rapid blood loss. When this occurs, blood flow to all the noncritical areas of the body—arms, legs, kidneys, liver, intestine—is shut off by the almost complete closure of blood vessels to those areas. The remaining blood supply is pumped to the two most critical areas which must have oxygen, the heart and the brain.

In the first stages of blood loss, the heart beats much more rapidly and squeezes harder in a desperate attempt to circulate the remaining blood more quickly. In addition, as already stated, blood vessels to all noncritical areas are shut down to maintain blood flow to the heart and brain. A person who loses blood quickly becomes cold as blood flow to the skin practically stops.

At a critical point, usually somewhere between 25 and 35 percent of rapid blood loss, blood pressure begins to fall rapidly. No matter how hard the heart tries, it cannot maintain adequate volume because of the continued loss of blood within this system. Just as in a water hose, the degree of pressure will determine how fast the fluid will flow. As the blood pressure drops, the blood flow decreases rapidly. With a drop in blood flow to critical areas of the brain, consciousness is quickly lost; if the problem is not resolved within minutes, death occurs. Death takes place in one of two ways: if the heart stops first, brain death will follow in three to five minutes. If the brain dies first, the heart will continue to pump as long as the blood it pumps supplies its own needs. (Remember that the heart is a muscle that needs its own blood supply to survive.)

Unless the blood loss is reversed by infusion of blood or fluids, the brain and heart may soon stop functioning because inadequate blood flow has caused infarction. Infarction indicates that an organ or part of an organ has been destroyed because of insufficient blood flow. When someone dies from blood loss, it is due to an infarction of either the heart or the brain. However, if one loses blood outside of the body, as from massive cuts, it may not be evident that the resulting heart attack or stroke was caused by blood loss itself rather than direct trauma. When a patient who has lost blood suffers a stroke or a heart attack, it is a common error to attribute this to the stress of the surgery or to the trauma itself when, in fact, the underlying cause may be the extreme degree of unreplaced blood loss.

A more logical explanation, in other words, is that the stroke or heart attack occurred because of insufficient perfusion of the brain or heart due to inadequate blood levels. The heart of a patient under-going surgery does not experience an increased workload the way the heart of a person who is exercising does. Nor is the heart usually subjected to increased activity or work during the postoperative pe-riod, when the patient simply lies in bed. Therefore, limited demands on the heart for increased work during and after surgery are, by themselves, unlikely to lead to a stroke or heart attack. On the other hand, inadequate blood or fluid replacement is very likely to result in diminished blood flow to those critical areas where a blood vessel has significant arteriosclerosis. In addition, if the heart is forced to oper-ate with thinned-out blood, it may have to work twice as hard as it would if missing blood had been fully replaced.

Changes in blood vessels are uneven: some blood vessels may be as unclogged as in youth, while others will show considerable narrow-ing. When blood replacement is inadequate, blood flow to certain constricted areas may fall below a critical threshold, so that the por-tion of the heart or brain involved may not be able to survive.

If the area involved is relatively small, the patient might have a small heart attack or stroke that goes entirely unnoticed by the pa-tient and his physician. If the area is large, then gross symptoms, such as chest pain in a heart attack or partial paralysis in a stroke, may ensue. Even more seriously, if the blood-starved area is in a critical portion of the heart or brain, sudden death may occur.

In most of these cases, the real, immediate cause of damage or death—namely, blood loss with inadequate blood replacement—may not be correctly identified. Instead, the patient will be diagnosed as having a stroke or heart attack. However, the cause of the heart attack may be mistakenly attributed to the surgery itself rather than to the inadequate replacement of blood.

Many small strokes and heart attacks are missed in the postoperative stage because patients frequently do not have follow-up cardiograms or special blood tests such as cardiac enzyme tests to diagnose these complications. The patient lying in bed may easily suffer a mild stroke that is completely overlooked by his physician, and that clears in a few days, yet nevertheless leaves some small, permanent damage.

In extreme cases when patients actually die, blood loss is usually not recognized as a possible cause. There is no way for a pathologist to determine the amount of blood a person has in his body at the time of death. It is even difficult to measure the exact amount of blood present in a living person. The pathologist will simply find that the patient had a form of stroke or heart attack without being able to recognize that the precipitating event was a grossly inadequate blood supply to the body.

BLOOD REPLACEMENT

The body can initially tolerate thinning of the blood better than the total absence of perfusion, or blood flow. In other words some blood, however thin, in every area of the body, is better than no blood at all in any one area.

When an area of the body receives no blood, it dies. Gangrene is a condition in which blood flow to a specific area has been cut off so that the affected part of the body cannot live. When blood is lost slowly, water and salts from other parts of the body are drawn into the bloodstream to dilute or thin out the remaining blood. In this way the body attempts to maintain a normal volume by providing a leaner mixture of blood to the body. It adjusts to the decrease in red cells by spreading them out more economically in diluted form.

As mentioned above, the rapid loss of one half or even 40 percent of blood volume will usually result in death. However, if the loss is gradual, it is possible for the body to lose one half of its red cells, or even more, while maintaining normal volume with thinned-out blood.

The body has a number of defenses that enable it to survive dramatic blood loss. Most important is the ability to provide water to maintain an adequate volume. In this way, at least some blood, however thin, can reach all parts of the body. Any area that does not have blood perfusion or a steady blood flow is at significantly greater risk. It is therefore understandable that, within certain limits, salt water can act as an adequate replacement for lost blood. The key question is, what are those limits, and what are the consequences of the current medical practice of replacing blood with water?

Under today's standard operating procedures, it is normal to replace blood loss of up to one third of volume—or three to four pints—with water. To understand the risks involved, recall that by FDA standards even a healthy person should donate no more than a single pint of blood every eight weeks. It is therefore quite contrary to sound physiological principles to claim that it is acceptable for people in their sixties and seventies to lose as much as four pints of blood after surgery and have it replaced only with sterile water. The loss of so much blood without an adequate replacement lowers both the hemoglobin and hematocrit levels and places the patient in significant danger of a major complication. Add to this the fact that doctors often unavoidably underestimate real blood loss, and the practice of substituting water for blood appears even more questionable.

It is relatively common in some hospitals for individuals to be missing half their red cells after cardiac surgery without receiving any additional blood replacement. It is claimed that these patients heal as well as if they had a full, normal supply. To appreciate the absurdity of such claims, compare two groups of patients. One group receives total blood replacement after surgery. The other group has only half of its red cells replaced. Which group has the better chance of recovery?

While no study has specifically targeted such groups, the *Lancet* findings suggest that hemoglobin levels and blood loss during surgery are important determinants of mortality.[23] When the hemoglobin falls below certain levels, the researchers recommend that doctors administer preoperative transfusions. Up to a point, the more blood a patient has before an operation and the less he loses during the procedure, the better are his chances for survival and recovery afterward.

The Yale study with animals also clearly demonstrates that bleeding an animal down to a 30 percent hematocrit level markedly lowers immunity.[24] Without a normal blood level, the animals became more susceptible to infection with poor healing. Animals have similar hematocrits to humans, with 45 percent being the norm. If animals show lower immunity and increased susceptibility to infection at a 30 percent hematocrit level, it is likely that people suffer similar reductions in immunity and disease-fighting capability at comparably low blood levels. It is imporant to note that the animals in the Yale study were only bled down and did not have to undergo the additional stress of surgery, as opposed to human patients who must bear the trauma of surgery while simultaneously being bled down to a hematocrit level of 30 percent or lower.

In human beings, simple calculation shows that lowering blood flow and blood-oxygen content by 50 percent in vessels that are already seriously compromised may lower oxygen below a critical level. Infarction and death of that portion of the organ involved are far more likely to occur under such circumstances.

Many people with heart disease who undergo a coronary angiography* are found to have some of their blood vessels as much as 90 percent closed off. Continued life in the affected portion of the heart literally hangs by a thread. When blood thins out beyond a critical point the oxygen supply falls below a critical level, and that portion of the heart muscle supplied by the narrowed blood vessels infarcts or dies. Clearly, replacement of normal blood levels is crucial to assure the best therapeutic results and to avoid such catastrophic events.

In the past three years, as AIDS has continued to spread, there has been a general movement among members of the medical profession to tolerate ever greater degrees of undertransfusion without blood replacement. The full extent of complications and fatalities resulting from this practice is rarely acknowledged. Instead, the complications are attributed to the patient's underlying problem. In the blood bank of the future, such deleterious practices will be greatly diminished.

---

*An angiography is an X-ray study of blood vessels where dye is injected into the vessel and reveals the degree of blockage.

8

The Blood Bank
of the Future

In health care facilities, all reasonable strategies to avoid a transfusion
of someone else's blood (homologous transfusion) should be
implemented by substituting, whenever possible, transfusion with
one's own blood (autologous transfusion).

Presidential Committee on the HIV Epidemic, June 1988

The safest blood is blood you've donated for yourself.

Dr. Lewellys Barker, senior vice president
of the American Red Cross, January 1989

B lood collected from a patient for retransfusion at a later time—
autologous blood—eliminates the risk of infection and immunologic reaction. You cannot give yourself AIDS, hepatitis, CMV, or any
other infectious disease nor can you have an allergic reaction to your
own blood. The use of one's own blood may also guard against the
dangers of immunosuppression associated with transfusions from
foreign donors.[1] Today everyone—the American Red Cross, the
American Association of Blood Banks, the Centers for Disease Control, the American Medical Association, the Food and Drug Administration—agrees that the safest blood is your own. Unfortunately, it
took the AIDS crisis to bring this self-evident fact to public awareness.

Considering the fact that it took 35 years for this scientific information to be publicly accepted, it is not surprising that another funda-

145

mental concept is still being denied by most members of the medical and blood banking establishment: namely, the obvious benefit of minimizing exposure to multiple donors and the advantages of donor selection. This chapter will consider how blood banking can and should be practiced in an ideal future setting *utilizing the techniques and tools that already exist.* The contrast with present practices should make it clear how far we have to go before achieving that ideal.

WHAT'S WRONG WITH MOST CURRENT AUTOLOGOUS TRANSFUSION PROGRAMS?

Clearly, it is illogical to expect to be able to donate blood to oneself just prior to needing it. As we have discussed, a person who needs a blood transfusion has already lost blood or is about to lose it. Such a person is hardly an ideal candidate for blood donation.

In fact, the most optimistic projection today is that only 10 percent of all individuals requiring a transfusion would actually have enough time to store some blood prior to surgery.[2] In other words, under the current method of autologous donation, only one out of ten patients would even theoretically have enough time to utilize this opportunity. However, as we shall see, even this figure is inflated and unrealistic when one considers the length of time it takes to make up the amount of blood donated just prior to surgery.

First, a great deal of so-called "elective surgery"—when people choose the place and time of surgery and so in theory can store their own blood ahead of time—is really semiemergency surgery and not truly elective. If an individual is suddenly discovered to have a malignant tumor, does he or she really want to wait four to six weeks to have the tumor removed so that there is enough time to store blood? Most people would prefer to have the tumor removed immediately.

A similar situation occurs with patients requiring cardiac bypass surgery. While many such patients know for months and even years that they have heart disease, the decision to undergo surgery is often very sudden, with less than ten days' preparation time. Such patients obviously do not have adequate time to store their own blood. At best, they can have a procedure called hemodilution—which, as will be shown in this chapter, has limited benefits.

We have already shown that withdrawing multiple units of blood in a short time is inadvisable since it frequently takes the body two to six weeks to make up a single unit. The older one is, the longer it takes to regenerate blood. This is the basis of the FDA rule that even healthy people should not donate more than once every eight weeks: the two-month recovery period gives individual donors adequate time to make up the loss of a single unit.*

When an individual donates multiple units within five weeks of surgery, his blood is in effect being diluted and he is weakened overall. The thinned-out blood cannot carry as much oxygen and, as a result, the heart must pump that much harder to deliver the same amount of oxygen. As stated previously, it is relatively common for a person who has just completed cardiac surgery to be missing half the red cells in her body and yet receive no further blood replacement. Clearly, the last thing a physician should want is a patient who must recuperate from heart surgery without half the red cells in her body. Yet this is a common occurrence today.

Instead of the optimistic 10 percent figure for people having adequate time to store blood for themselves prior to needing it, in reality probably less than 5 percent of all transfusion recipients could safely predonate their own blood. This is because fewer than 5 percent have enough time to replace their donated blood before surgery. Consequently, for 95 percent of the people who need blood, the concept of autologous donation as currently practiced—donating blood to oneself just prior to needing it—has limited practical value, and it may actually put some patients at greater risk than if no blood were taken before surgery. Realistically, to expect to be able to donate blood just before needing it makes about as much sense as expecting to be able to put your seat belt on in the middle of an accident.

One hopes that it will not take another 35 years before the medical and blood banking establishment acknowledges that *the safest amount of blood to have in a medical or surgical emergency is a full quantity of one's own blood.* It is medically unjustified to claim that individuals missing one-third to one-half of the red cells in their body do not need these red cells during and after surgery—and that they can recover as well as individuals with a normal supply of blood and normal clotting factors. Individuals should only become blood donors for themselves when there is adequate time to avoid becoming anemic; and they

*Organizations like the American Red Cross recommend that healthy subjects donate no more than five times, or five units of blood, in one year. Yet for predonation autologous programs—and for patients facing surgery—the Red Cross, along with the AABB, supports the practice of donating up to five units of blood within five weeks.

should donate only as much blood as can be taken without significant thinning of their own blood. Individuals should *not* become blood donors for themselves, nor lose blood without replacement, prior to the rigors of an operation and the stresses of the postoperative period unless there is adequate time for regeneration of the donated blood.

It is hard to believe that a person missing three pints of blood after surgery would be denied retransfusion with his own blood from a hospital blood bank. Unfortunately, this is occurring today in a number of cases and without the patients' consent or knowledge. Some patients with hematocrits slightly above 33 percent—which means, in effect, that they may be missing almost three pints of their own red cells—are not receiving blood they had previously donated and stored for themselves. Instead the blood is given to other, even more anemic patients with the justification that someone with a 33 percent hematocrit doesn't really need more blood. What these patients are not being told is that they are really missing two or more pints of blood and that they have effectively been converted into involuntary blood donors for someone else.

I know of one case in which a woman, after delivering her baby, bled down to a hematocrit of 31 percent. Instead of transfusing the woman with her own blood, which she had predonated and which was waiting for her in the hospital blood bank, the doctors discharged her without giving her any blood. The woman left the hospital in a markedly weakened state, missing between two and three pints of blood— yet reassured by her physicians that she was fine and did not need any blood at all. Her blood was then given to another patient.*

These practices violate every patient's basic right to be treated with the safest medical and surgical procedures available. No patient missing *any* amount of blood after surgery should be denied retransfusion with his own blood when it is available on the grounds that he does not really need it. No hospital should give an anemic patient's blood to another patient without written consent. Patients should insist that they get their own blood back and that they be transfused to a full, normal level. It is unjustified to use the same low, minimal transfu-

---

*It is not surprising that women are often weak after childbirth, since they not infrequently lose between one quarter and one third of their blood during delivery— in a regular vaginal delivery, as well as in a cesarean section. If there is one definitive situation where an individual has adequate warning prior to blood use, it is pregnancy. Every woman contemplating childbirth or in the early stages of pregnancy should store her own blood.

sion guidelines—a hematocrit level of 30 percent—for patients who have their own safe blood available as for those patients who must rely on the general blood supply and thus face significantly higher risks. Any patient who has stored her own blood in advance should have free and full access to this safe source of transfusion. No hospital or physician should have the right to block a patient from having access to her own blood when it is available from a federally licensed blood bank. Nor should any patient recovering from surgery be made an involuntary donor for another—certainly not without his full knowledge and permission. Each patient should have the right to use his own blood when available and select his own donor. And every patient must be free to take steps to minimize the number of donors to which he is exposed.

There is a lawsuit in New Jersey, currently pending, concerning a patient who contracted AIDS from a blood transfusion and is suing the hospital, the blood bank, and the physicians for violating the basic rights just enumerated.[3] Four weeks before surgery, this patient asked to store his own blood and select his own donors. The hospital refused, and the patient subsequently underwent cardiac surgery, where he contracted AIDS from a transfusion. Yet despite the magnitude of the injury, the patient discovered that he could sue the hospital for only $10,000, which is the limit in New Jersey for any lawsuit filed against a nonprofit hospital. Most individuals who sue hospitals and doctors after developing AIDS or hepatitis from a blood transfusion discover that the system is stacked against them and that they have no legal recourse. Meanwhile, blood banking organizations have successfully lobbied federal and state legislatures for special laws that protect them from gross misrepresentation and negligence.

A cardiac surgeon who tells a patient that his chances of dying from an operation are 1 in 10,000 when the real risk might be 1 in 50, could easily be sued. Similarly, any hospital, doctor, or blood bank claiming today that is extremely rare to develop an infection from a blood transfusion—when the infection rate is at least between 5 and 10 percent per patient—is guilty of fraudulent representation. Until recently, however, patients misled about the risks of a blood transfusion were unaware they had any right to object. The current spate of lawsuits against the blood industry may finally compel all hospitals and blood banks to operate under the principle of informed consent: every transfusion recipient, like every other patient, will have the right to know the true risks of the medical or surgical procedure about to be carried out. It is most regrettable that such improvements in medical practice must result from attacks by injured parties and their lawyers, and not from positive changes within the system itself.

Today many concerned members of the public believe that safe methods of autologous transfusion are available as an alternative to standard blood transfusions. It is true that self-storage of blood has doubled in each of the last two years, and that multiple facilities now offer some form of autologous donation in response to growing public concern about the safety of the blood supply. However, with the exception of frozen blood programs, current autologous services consist of three basic techniques, all of which have major limitations.

Intraoperative salvage, for example, is a good way of recapturing some of the blood that is spilled in the operative field during surgry. Most of this blood cannot be recovered, but even a 10 to 25 percent recovery does reduce the need for additional transfusion. Therefore, intraoperative salvage is a useful tool for transfusion therapy and a positive development in the field. In this process, the patient's lost blood is collected ("salvaged"), washed, and reinfused as soon as possible through a machine sometimes known as a "cell saver." However, as just noted, most of the blood lost during an operation cannot be recovered with this technique.[4] Furthermore, patients frequently continue to suffer internal blood loss for several days after recovery, and intraoperative salvage can be used only during open surgery. For all its benefits, intraoperative salvage has basic limitations.

A similar technique, known as postoperative salvage, is used to recapture profuse blood lost after open heart surgery and traumatic hemothorax. It employs the same devices for collecting and filtering blood that are used during surgery. Postoperative salvage does not improve a patient's coagulation status—the blood collected is defibrinogenated and will not clot—but in certain cases it does reduce somewhat the number of red blood cell transfusions required. However, since the clotting elements cannot be salvaged, a patient may also need additional transfusions of plasma and platelets.

A third technique, hemodilution, is a popular variant of autologous transfusion in which the blood is thinned out and replaced with salt water in the last few hours before surgery. The blood collected during hemodilution is saved and retransfused later. The primary aim of the procedure is to have a safe supply of the patient's own (thinned-out) blood available for transfusion. The other aim is to reduce the workload on the heart during surgery—since the blood is thin and has less viscosity—and so facilitate the circulation. However, as we saw earlier, decreasing the oxygen-carrying capacity of the blood forces the heart to work that much harder to deliver the same amount of oxygen. The slight decrease in work created by reducing the viscosity or "stickiness" of the blood is far outweighed by the extra work the heart must do to pump more thinned-out blood in order to oxygenate the body adequately.

Some physicians and blood bankers now recommend hemodilution as a way of avoiding a transfusion. Under certain circumstances, patients may actually succeed in avoiding the transfusion, but there is a significant increase in their exposure to other risks.* Patients undergoing hemodilution are bled down and replaced with salt water betweeen six and two hours before their surgery. This procedure dilutes their blood and lowers its oxygen-carrying capacity; as a result, blood flow and oxygen delivery to a partially blocked coronary or cerebral artery may be decreased just enough to precipitate a stroke or heart attack. Keep in mind that almost all individuals over 50 years have some variable decrease in their coronary and cerebral arteries. Pumping thinned-out blood through a partially clogged artery may tip the balance toward destruction of a portion of the brain or heart served by that artery.

Once again, a primary objective of hemodilution is to avoid giving a potentially dangerous transfusion with someone else's blood. Unfortunately such evasive measures may result in greater damage to the patient. In point of fact, much of the current presurgical autologous transfusion is simply disguised hemodilution: an individual is bled multiple times and his blood is thinned out over a period of weeks rather than hours.

In standard "predeposit" transfusion, patients facing surgery donate blood for themselves in the five weeks prior to an operation. However, as we have seen, 90 to 95 percent of all surgical patients are simply not in a position to predonate blood before needing it. Those who do qualify for presurgical donation often make themselves anemic and blood-depleted prior to an operation, thus jeopardizing their chances of recovery. If one were to allow predonation autologous transfusion only to those patients who have adequate time to replace their blood *before* surgery—as any rational medical policy should—at

---

*Because they have higher initial hematocrits (45 percent), men are better candidates for mild hemodilution than women (39 percent). Women who have not stored blood are at significantly greater risk with respect to having adequate time to store blood and avoid anemia. A woman who loses an amount of blood equal to a man will become significantly anemic before a man reaches the same state of anemia.

least half of the donors currently considered eligible for autologous transfusion would be eliminated. All anemic and blood-depleted individuals would be barred from predonating their own blood, leaving an eligible patient pool of less than 5 percent. Thus 95 percent of those who need a transfusion do not really have adequate warning to donate ahead of time and still make up their blood prior to surgery.

In order to avoid creating anemia and blood depletion in patients about to undergo surgery, blood should be obtained only from individuals who have enough time to make up their lost blood prior to surgery. This would mean at least a two-week waiting period for most forms of surgery, since few individuals can make up an extra pint in less than two weeks. It would also set a practical donor limit of about two pints prior to surgery, since only a few individuals could make up more than two pints within the six-week lifespan of refrigerated blood.

While there have been some advances in autologous blood transfusion practices, what passes for "safe" self-storage of blood today is, in fact, unavailable for more than 90 percent of those requiring a transfusion and presents a significant risk for the remaining 5 to 10 percent for whom it is advocated. The three techniques outlined above can only meet the needs of a small fraction of patients requiring blood transfusions each year. There is, however, a clear and simple way to get one's own safe blood in the event one needs it or, at a minimum, to get a much safer form of blood than is currently available and to minimize donor exposure and donor risk.

FROZEN AUTOLOGOUS BLOOD

Everyone understands that you do not buy fire insurance when your house is burning down. Neither should you expect to be able to obtain adequate blood insurance after you are ill or injured. Like most such policies, blood insurance protection involves adequate planning and preparation prior to the development of an urgent problem.

Since the studies of pioneers like Drs. Charles Huggins, Arthur Rowe, Edmund Valeri, and H. T. Meryman, it has been known that by utilizing special techniques blood can be stored for as long as 20 years. The American Red Cross, despite publicly frowning on frozen autologous blood, has itself been freezing blood since 1964. In 1987, the FDA officially extended the storage period for frozen blood from 3 to 10 years. There is little doubt that the 20-year storage period will ultimately be approved, as documentation already exists that blood can be safely stored for transfusion purposes for this length of time.[5] Both the blood plasma, which contains the clotting factors, and the cellular components—chiefly the red cells—can be effectively frozen. (Platelets at the present time do not freeze as well.)

An individual can safely store his or her own blood at intervals of eight weeks or more and so build up a personal blood supply in the event of a medical or surgical emergency. This procedure totally avoids the risks associated with donating multiple units of blood prior to surgery.

In many medical situations such as kidney disease, pneumonia, and medication reactions, an individual may gradually lose blood. Such an individual may not require surgery but may nevertheless require a blood transfusion. Obviously this person has no chance of receiving his or her own blood unless it was stored well in advance. A large percentage of patients who receive transfusions need them for such reasons and not for operations. These patients, who are already blood-depleted, could only receive their own blood if they had stored it ahead of time, before their medical problems began. The majority of transfusions are given to such people who are already blood-depleted and who are in no position to donate to themselves or anyone else when they discover that they will need a transfusion.

When we bleed, we lose whole blood. Frequently, however, only the red cells are initially replaced by transfusion. There are two reasons cited as justification for not immediately replacing plasma: first, it involves certain risks of its own; and second, one does not need plasma until the clotting factors in the blood are reduced to dangerous levels.

Although what constitutes a dangerous level is a matter of medical conjecture, clearly the best level of clotting factors to have is a normal one, not one diminished by 30 or 40 or even 50 percent. Hemophilia is a disease in which one of the blood clotting factors (Factor VIII) is present in inadequate quantity, a deficiency that causes recurrent bleeding. The standard tests for blood clotting are performed in test tubes and are designed to imitate the conditions in the body. Unfortunately, these tests are merely estimates and cannot absolutely duplicate a bleeding situation in the body in which hundreds of small capillaries may have been cut. With this in mind, we can see that it is certainly no advantage to be missing as much as 50 percent or more of one's clotting elements, as is frequently the case when plasma is not transfused.

However, if one stores blood in advance, one does not have to be deprived of plasma until significant bleeding has taken place. With frozen self-storage, whole blood—plasma and all—is available, instead of the usual skimmed blood with no plasma.

There are probably a significant number of cases in which people bleed longer than necessary because they receive multiple red cell transfusions without adequate replacement of plasma, which contains the clotting factors. Since the current practice is to use a separate donor for plasma, for platelets, and for red cells, the reluctance of physicians to give plasma is somewhat understandable. Simple arithmetic shows that if one receives plasma and red cells from the same donor, one immediately and significantly reduces the risk of infection and immunologic reaction. Yet almost no effort is currently made to supply plasma and red cells from the same donor.

There are specific advantages to frozen blood. Blood kept in a liquid, refrigerated state ages (the longest that refrigerated blood can be used is 42 days), while frozen blood cells remain fresh almost indefinitely. Frozen cells also retain special enzymes that are lost when blood is stored in a refrigerated nonfrozen state for more than a week.

In the standard practice of blood bank management programs, the oldest blood is always given to patients first in order to avoid outdating and to conserve supplies. This practice—similar to the grocer's practice of keeping the oldest milk and butter up front—is a good one from the management point of view, but it is not necessarily good from the patient's perspective, since the fresher the blood, the more effective it is for the patient.

The average transfused blood cell is already 60 days old. Normal healthy blood cells live only 120 days within the body. New red blood cells are constantly being made because of the daily average loss of 1 percent. Since the natural life span of a blood cell is 120 days at most, receiving a transfusion from blood that has been stored almost 42 days means that these cells will survive a significantly shorter time than if they had been stored only 1 or 2 days.

By contrast, blood frozen within 24 hours and kept frozen for two years is fresher than blood that has been kept refrigerated for 35 days. This is because blood maintained in a proper, superfrozen state barely ages. After two years, the loss in the number of stored, frozen red cells—usually between 5 and 10 percent—will be *less* than the loss of red cells from blood that has been refrigerated for 35 days.[6] Freezing blood arrests the process of aging and deterioration.

When we talk about freezing blood, we obviously do not mean simply popping it into the freezer. Freezing blood directly will destroy it. It took several decades of research and contributions from many individual researchers to devise the various techniques used to enable blood to survive temperatures between 150° and 350° Fahrenheit below the freezing point. At these superlow temperatures, blood must be mixed with a special type of preservative or antifreeze that enables the blood cells to survive.

The cryopreservative, or antifreeze, is a special compound that is mixed with the blood to prevent the cells from being destroyed when they are frozen. Glycerol, which removes water from the cells and limits ice formation, is the most common additive used. Special techniques are required to mix the blood with glycerol—the most delicate part of the procedure—as well as to freeze it at a rate that avoids injury to the cells.

There are several subtle variations that ensure the almost complete recovery of the blood cells. These techniques should be used only by an expert in freezing technology, as there are many stages where an error can render the frozen blood useless. Just as in any technological procedure, good technique and good technicians are essential.

When the blood is thawed in special chambers, the preservative must be removed or deglycerolized in a series of steps. The process of thawing and separating the preservative so that blood is ready for transfusion takes approximately 45 minutes to an hour. New methods of thawing may shorten this period to 10 minutes.

Blood is normally kept frozen at −120° Fahrenheit (−80° Centigrade), or 217° Fahrenheit below body temperature. The process of thawing requires bringing the frozen blood back to the liquid state by immersion in a special water bath kept at body temperature. After the blood is thawed, the use of specially designed equipment enables the preservative to be removed without breaking sterility. The blood is usually brought up to a temperature a few degrees above freezing and shipped in a refrigerated state to a hospital or wherever it is needed.

Depending upon the method used, it takes about an hour to prepare a unit of frozen blood so that it is ready for shipment. In the New York metropolitan area, blood can be delivered anywhere within two hours—and is, every day—using motorized couriers. Emergency couriers can deliver blood within a 45 mile radius inside of 75 minutes. The blood can be transfused shortly after arriving.

Nevertheless, many people are under the erroneous impression that frozen blood will not be delivered in time, particularly if they are in a car accident or some other emergency far from home. This is an extremely unlikely scenario and a thoroughly unjustified concern. It is based on the very common misperception—fostered to some degree by television drama and the movies—that an injured person rushed to a hospital emergency room begins receiving blood right away. In practice, blood transfusions are rarely given to *anyone*, including accident victims, within the first six hours of hospitalization; fewer than 5 percent of all transfusions are given to patients within six hours of admission. In the most comprehensive survey of this kind to date, doctors at Cedars of Sinai Hospital in California found that only 23 out of 1,156 transfusion recipients—or only about 2 percent—needed blood in the first four hours.[7]

In addition, fewer than 12 percent of *all* transfusions are given for trauma such as car accidents. Most transfusions are given for medical and surgical reasons unrelated to trauma. In other words, if you are unfortunate enough to require a blood transfusion, the chances are 9 out of 10 that you were *not* in a traumatic accident. Furthermore, if you *are* injured in an emergency, statistically the most likely place to have an accident is in your home or neighborhood, not at the opposite end of the country.

The typical person who needs a blood transfusion is someone who has bled over a period of time before he becomes so ill that he is admitted to the hospital. Many patients, including surgical patients, actually receive a limited amount of blood within the first 24 hours and additional blood one or more days after the problem is treated. A patient who is hospitalized with blood loss will routinely receive salt water replacement until his blood level is stabilized and some estimate made of the amount of blood lost. Transfusions, therefore, are almost never initiated within the first six hours of admission. Frequently it takes longer, and the first transfusion, even after significant blood loss, may not be given for 24 hours.

Today, with the widespread recognition of the dangers of blood transfusion, and the fear engendered by AIDS, most hospitals deliberately delay transfusions as long as they can unless pressed by an absolute need. Therefore, as it stands now, even if you are in an accident and are willing to accept blood from the general supply, you will probably not receive any blood for at least six hours and then only after you have lost massive amounts. However, if you have stored your own blood and are unlucky enough to be in a car accident—even at the opposite end of the country—the chances are excellent that you will get your own blood in time.

Blood can be shipped by special courier anywhere in the country through the quickest combination of surface and air transport available. In November 1988, the company with which I am affiliated signed an agreement with Federal Express. This agreement calls for a national center in Memphis where stored blood can be delivered anywhere in the United States within an average period of six hours. Other autologous blood banks, such as Hemacare in California, can provide similar services on a regional basis.

In a recent case of mine, a young lady fractured her leg in a car accident in Maryland. She was rushed to the local hospital, where she received the usual salt water replacement for blood. Over a 24-hour period, she lost over half the blood in her body, yet all she received in replacement was salt water. Finally, the decision was made to transfuse the patient with blood. Her father, a New York executive, had not yet stored his own blood but fortunately had arranged for his two office assistants to do so. One of the assistants, who had stored two pints of frozen blood, had the same blood type as his daughter.

Within an hour, this blood was ready for emergency courier service. It was rushed to La Guardia airport, where it was flown to Washington, D.C., and delivered via courier to Maryland. Within three hours of shipment, the blood was at the patient's hospital and ready for cross-matching and transfusion.

This particular patient, who received two pints of whole blood (two units apiece of red cells and plasma) was thus exposed to one known donor as opposed to four unknown donors. Even if one assumes that the father's office assistant was no "safer" than a donor from the general population, simply by limiting the number of donors, the patient had reduced her risk by 75 percent. Over a number of days, this patient's condition stabilized. Eventually she received three more units of blood from her family and underwent successful surgery.

By instituting a system of regional, frozen blood centers able to ship blood within 2 to 6 hours, one could meet the needs of over 90 percent of blood transfusion recipients whether they were facing a medical or a surgical situation. In this patient's case, even if she had been in California, she could easily have received her own blood from New York within 12 hours.

We therefore maintain that the overwhelming majority of those individuals who have stored frozen blood will be able to have their own blood delivered to them in a timely fashion. Indeed, in the four years since we opened the first public autologous blood bank, there has not been *a single case* when someone needed stored blood—either for himself or for a friend or relative—but could not get it in time and was thus forced to take blood from an unknown donor. Obviously such cases will occur, but they represent only a small fraction of all the blood transfusions that are administered.

Another common objection to an autologous system is that if people begin to store blood for themselves, there won't be enough blood for the community. The notion that frozen autologous blood storage is selfish is misleading. This negative attitude has been propagated by organizations such as the Red Cross that depend on voluntary donations to obtain their blood supply. Many of these organizations wrongly fear that the storage of blood by individuals for themselves and their families will somehow cut into the available blood supply for the general public. Actually, the need for blood is so great that there would be no diminution in voluntary blood banking activities if a frozen, autologous system were also adopted. In fact, self-storage of blood will help to alleviate present blood shortages. Many regions of the country now function with only a one- or two-day supply of blood. During holidays and summer vacations there are frequently acute shortages and frantic appeals to the public. The New York Blood Center, the single largest blood bank in the country, must import over 25 percent of its blood from abroad. We would consider it unacceptable to operate with a two-day national food supply, nor would we tolerate a two-day national oil supply; why tolerate a two-day blood supply?* These chronic blood shortages will only be remedied by a frozen blood supply system. In addition, by encouraging individuals to store blood for themselves, we will ensure that they are not a drain on the existing blood supply.

There are other benefits to a frozen autologous program. Fewer than 4 percent of the population now donate blood each year for the remaining 96 percent. Many people are either afraid of giving blood or have never been sufficiently motivated to go to a blood bank. Once these people undergo the experience of donating for themselves, they may actually be more inclined to donate for the general supply. In fact, people who have stored blood for themselves often end by releasing it for the benefit of others. In the Daxor autologous blood program, over 50 percent of the blood that has already been used—

---

*Often today there is a one-day and even zero-day blood supply, necessitating that some surgery be delayed or canceled.

blood originally stored by individuals for themselves—was ultimately used for relatives and friends or released into the general blood supply rather than being used for the original donor. While some of these autologous donors were primarily concerned about themselves and their families in the event of a blood emergency, their actions helped to alleviate the general blood shortage.

With the wider use of frozen blood, there will be a healthy interface between the voluntary and private sectors. Private, frozen blood stores will act as a buffer against sudden shortages. In a public emergency, many people would be more willing, and more likely, to donate from their private supply of blood than to make a special trip to the blood bank for this purpose. Rather than compounding a problem that already exists, the advent of frozen, autologous blood may once and for all wipe out the chronic shortages of blood that repeatedly threaten the American blood supply.

DONATING BLOOD AHEAD OF TIME: HOW, AND HOW MUCH?

Most individuals would not consider driving in an uninsured car. Yet some people may eventually require a blood transfusion as a result of an accident involving that car. An uninsured car may bring about a financial loss; a transfusion with infected blood may result in a loss of life. Therefore if one has a choice between car and blood insurance, one should choose the latter. In the blood bank of the future, every family will have such insurance.

When Daxor, the company with which I am affiliated, established the first long-term autologous blood bank in the United States, and in the world, the following guidelines were agreed upon: (a) blood can be taken from anyone who is not anemic regardless of age, with the exact amount determined by health and body size, and (b) the frequency with which blood can be taken is determined by health. These guidelines work out well for the elderly, who may require more than two months to replenish blood safely; under a frozen autologous system they could safely store two units over a 1-year period.* These

---

*It is never too late to store blood. In a recently reported medical case a 90-year-old man was infected with AIDS from a blood transfusion he received when he was 85. In our blood program we have had a 93-year-old man store blood for himself with no difficulty by taking a few simple, extra precautions.

units would then be viable for up to 20 years. Thus, elderly patients would not have to risk anemia by predonating blood in the weeks prior to an operation; nor, if they lost much blood during surgery, would they have to remain undertransfused because of the risk of infection.

Relying on relatives to donate blood at the time of an emergency is risky, for blood is not simply withdrawn from one person's vein and injected into another's. At most blood banks it now takes three to five days to complete all the tests necessary to prepare blood for transfusion. If you can afford to wait that long when you need a transfusion, and if your relative is immediately on hand with the same blood type as you, then this delay will present no problem (although even with relatives donating fresh, unfrozen blood, there is no guarantee that these donors are free of AIDS, since there is not enough time to retest them). On the other hand, there is the possibility that you can wait no more than 6 to 24 hours for a transfusion. In that case, even having a relative on hand with your blood type is no guarantee that you will be able to avoid getting the blood you need from any anonymous donor instead of from someone you have selected. However, if your relative had stored blood in a frozen state, that blood would have been previously tested and available for transfusion within several hours instead of several days.

Most people assume they can rely on the national blood banking system to meet any need in an emergency. In fact, the one thing you can be virtually sure of is that you *won't* get all the blood you need for complete replacement when you lose blood unless you store it for yourself. Unless you take personal responsibility for your own blood needs and those of your family, you will be subject to the present policy of undertransfusion and inadequate replacement of blood. Alternatively, if you have your own frozen stored blood available, proper full replacement can take place. A doctor who knows that you have stored your own risk-free blood should not hesitate to provide you with complete replacement when you lose blood.*

Under ideal conditions an individual should not be left missing

---

*Physicians have been so accustomed to the danger of communicating disease through blood transfusion that it may take some time for them to get reoriented to the idea that patients should have complete replacement when their own safe blood is available. For this reason, it is imperative that patients discuss these matters with their physician in advance. Several recent studies have shown that the mere fact of having one's own autologous blood on hand alters the attitude and behavior of physicians in a positive way.[8]

more than one pint of blood, for the danger of a major complication increases geometrically with each pint of blood that is not replaced. If one loses four pints of blood, one has a much higher risk than an individual who has lost two pints. Someone who has lost six pints has an extremely high chance of not surviving the experience without some blood replacement. To guard against such possibilities, even a single unit of your own stored blood provides significant protection. You might lose as much as one-third of your blood and have two units replaced with sterile water and only one with blood and still be relatively safe. Moreover, storage of one pint coupled with some units from a close blood relative does provide a reasonable margin of safety in many situations when blood is needed. Thus, even one pint of stored blood can make a crucial difference to the consequences of blood loss.

Though it is possible to have safe blood available for ready use by storing blood at a time when there is no anticipated need for it, some poeple wonder how such a program would actually work out in terms of age, health, body size, et cetera.

The fact is that anyone can donate blood, including children, as long as they are not in an anemic or blood-depleted state. A healthy person weighing more than 110 pounds can easily donate one pint. Smaller people or young children can store blood for themselves by simply having smaller amounts of blood removed in proportion to their body size (in Japan, it is common for individuals to donate half a pint instead of a full pint because of their smaller size). A normal American adult has between 8 and 12 pints of blood, depending on body size. Women, being relatively smaller, tend to have less blood than men, as Table 2 shows. Readers may use this table to determine their individual blood volume by locating their height and weight and finding the corresponding figure inside the table. This figure gives normal blood volume, expressed in pints. Thus a man who is five feet, eight inches tall and weighs 160 pounds has about 10.8 pints of blood in his body. A woman who is five feet, eight inches tall and weighs 160 pounds has about 10.1 pints of blood in her body. When persons of approximately this size donate one pint of blood, they are donating about 10 percent of their total blood volume.

Another important question concerns the practicality of a frozen blood program from the point of view of cost. The following examples are taken from our own experience.

A reasonable, minimal blood program for a family of four (two adults and two children) would be to have the two adults store at least

Table 2   Normal Blood Volume (Pints) According to Height and Weight

	Men, Weight (lb)										
Height	120	130	140	150	160	170	180	190	200	210	220
5'2"	8.8	9.0	9.1	9.3	9.5	9.7	10	10.3	10.6	10.9	11.1
5'4"	9.2	9.4	9.6	9.7	9.9	10.1	10.3	10.6	10.9	11.2	11.5
5'6"	9.7	9.9	10.1	10.2	10.3	10.5	10.7	10.9	11.2	11.5	11.8
5'8"	10.1	10.3	10.5	10.7	10.8	10.9	11.1	11.3	11.6	11.8	12.1
5'10"	10.6	10.8	11.0	11.2	11.3	11.5	11.6	11.8	12	12.2	12.5
6'0"	10.8	11.1	11.3	11.5	11.6	11.8	11.9	12.1	12.3	12.5	12.7
6'2"	11.1	11.4	11.6	11.8	12	12.2	12.3	12.4	12.6	12.8	13
6'4"	11.5	11.8	12.1	12.4	12.6	12.7	12.9	13	13.1	13.2	13.5

	Women, Weight (lb)								
Height	100	110	120	130	140	150	160	170	180
4'10"	7.3	7.4	7.6	7.9	8	8.3	8.6	8.9	9.2
5'0"	7.6	7.8	7.9	8.1	8.3	8.5	8.8	9.1	9.4
5'2"	7.9	8.1	8.3	8.4	8.6	8.8	9.1	9.3	9.6
5'4"	8.4	8.5	8.7	8.9	9	9.2	9.4	9.7	9.9
5'6"	8.7	9.0	9.1	9.3	9.5	9.6	9.8	10	10.3
5'8"	9.1	9.4	9.6	9.7	9.9	10	10.1	10.4	10.6
5'10"	9.4	9.7	10	10.3	10.2	10.5	10.6	10.7	11
6'0"	9.6	10	10.3	10.5	10.6	10.8	11	11.1	11.3

one pint of red cells each. Today one pint of red cells can be stored for $12 a month after an initial testing and processing fee of about $100. In most but not all instances, the children would likely cross-match with at least one parent. A pint of blood stored by an adult would be equivalent to two pints stored for a child because a child has a much smaller total blood volume. A child who weighs 65 pounds has four pints of blood, or half the volume of an adult weighing 130 pounds. Through appropriate use of the parents' stored blood, it may thus be unnecessary for the child to store any blood, allowing the family to have minimal coverage at a reasonable cost.

   Where cost is not a factor, then storing two or three pints of blood per individual would be preferable. With three pints of one's own blood in storage, one is equipped to handle the overwhelming majority of medical and surgical emergencies. Any individual with this kind of blood insurance can be confident of proper protection.

What if one needs more blood but cannot afford the cost of full personal coverage? By combining with other prescreened relatives or friends to form joint blood groups, one can establish additional sources through an exchange program. An individual who participates in such a group may have the benefit of blood coverage at a lower cost. One client at our blood bank with type O blood stored two pints for himself. He then designated 15 members of his family whose blood was compatible with his as potential recipients for his blood. In the event of an illness or injury to any of these people, they would have had a safe supply of blood immediately ready for transfusion. The cost to each of these family members for two pints of safe blood was less than $2 a person per month.

If plasma is also stored, which I strongly recommend, there is a separate, additional charge. A single unit of plasma for one person now costs about $8 a month to store or just under $100 a year. Most autologous blood banks do not store plasma—instead, they sell it. To guarantee maximum safety, however, everyone should also store some of his or her own plasma.

The ideal, maximum blood insurance for an individual today could thus cost as much as $60 a month. This would cover the storage of three units of red cells and three units of plasma, enough safe blood to meet most contingencies. This amount of blood, for example, would be adequate to compensate for the loss of more than half of an individual's entire blood supply. Storing two units of red cells and two units of plasma, at a cost of $40 a month, would also provide substantial protection.

Family and group coverage as outlined above can keep these costs at a reasonable level. For a family of four utilizing cross-coverage, maximum protection could be obtained for as little as $15 a member per month. While this cost is still high for the majority of Americans, economies of scale will eventually lower storage costs as the concept of frozen autologous blood storage develops and spreads.

In weighing the costs of a frozen autologous blood program, one should consider the much higher social costs of serious illness resulting from transfusion with unsafe blood. The average case of AIDS costs society between $100,000 and $200,000 in direct and indirect medical care, not to mention the incalculable cost from lost productivity and premature loss of life. The overall cost to society of care for AIDS patients and hepatitis victims is rapidly escalating into billions of dollars.* A single AIDS baby who lives in a hospital for one year now costs society over $300,000. The 4,000 new AIDS babies in 1988 will thus cost $1.2 billion. Surely we can justify a comparable investment in a new blood banking system that will help prevent these tragedies, and others, from occurring in the first place. A fully developed frozen blood storage system would more than pay for itself in savings to society at large.

There are, of course, the very poor who cannot afford any fees at all. Under the present system, medical services such as dialysis machines, prescription eyeglasses, and dental work are covered by Medicaid. As the need for frozen blood storage becomes more widely accepted, the social safety net will have to extend its coverage to this vital storage program. The provision of a safe blood supply for all members of society ought to be seen as a fundamental public health obligation.

Some forward-looking companies are already beginning to offer blood banking services as a benefit for employers. In 1987 Warner Communications, the film and records giant, became the first major company in the United States to provide frozen blood storage services for all its employees. Under the Warner program, employees now pay as little as $3 a month for blood storage. Other large companies and corporations will surely follow, if only to remain competitive.

It is my own opinion that the American Red Cross itself will eventually rethink its opposition to a private frozen autologous blood program. Once the present, self-serving, and patently false objections to frozen blood are publicly dispelled—and the temporary cost and inconvenience of switching systems is overcome—there is likely to be a full integration of the current voluntary and self-storage blood banking systems. Such a system will ultimately lead to a vast improvement in solving both the serious hazards now plaguing the blood supply and the problem of major blood shortages.

In 1989, the Pentagon kicked off the world's largest frozen blood program, a five-year project to draw 45,000 pints a year with the ultimate goal of stockpiling 225,000 pints domestically and abroad for use during combat or disaster. This ambitious program may well

---

*The American business community is unprepared for the full impact of these impending costs. See my article entitled "AIDS and Ostriches" in *Barrons*, December 18, 1989.

serve as a forerunner of more widespread civilian efforts to freeze and store safe blood.

The concept of frozen autologous blood banks has also caught the attention of the Japanese. With one of the highest hepatitis rates in the world, and an alarming incidence of HTLV-I in the densely populated south, Japan is particularly vulnerable to blood-borne diseases. After several exploratory visits, a number of Japanese executives have recently contracted with our company to develop the first autologous blood bank in Japan.

Additional sums to provide for safer blood and self-storage of blood are essential to guarantee the best medical care available in the United States. While there would be an initial increase in expenditure for a frozen autologous blood program, this would eventually be offset by the huge social savings from the prevention of serious illness. By way of comparison, consider that the cost of a single nuclear power plant, such as the Shoreham plant now being abandoned by New York State, exceeds the total cost of setting up a safe blood banking system for the entire United States. Surely there are better ways of spending public money.

The question we must ask is not whether we can afford such a program but whether we can afford *not* to have one, given the proven benefits in avoiding diseases and the guaranteed, tremendous saving of human life.

LIMITING DONOR EXPOSURE:
PLATELETS AND THE MONODONOR CONCEPT

When one bleeds, red cells, plasma, and platelets are lost. All these elements must be replaced or regenerated. It is not uncommon for individuals to get a disproportionate amount of one component or another in a transfusion, and in many situations patients are satisfactorily treated with red cells alone or with a varying combination of red cells and plasma.

Not infrequently, however, patients who have lost significant quantities of blood and been replaced only with red cell and plasma transfusions suddenly develop very low platelet counts. When people bleed, the bone marrow, where platelets—a key clotting agent—are made, is often suppressed. As the platelet count drops, the patient may experience a vicious cycle where he or she continues to bleed because the clots formed are inadequate to stop the bleeding due to the low platelets. (To understand the importance of platelets, consider how inadequate a brick wall would be if there were no mortar between the bricks to hold them together: the platelets hold the clot together in much the same way.)

In many cases patients persist in bleeding despite multiple transfusions because only partial transfusions, containing red cells alone, are given. Under these circumstances it is not uncommon for individuals suddenly to require between five and ten packs of platelets in a single transfusion. Since each pack contains the amount of platelets skimmed or separated from a single pint of donor blood, a five-pack transfusion contains platelets from five separate donors. And since a single platelet pack is as capable of producing AIDS or hepatitis as the red cells or plasma from which it has been separated, a patient who receives five or ten packs of platelets in one transfusion has suddenly been exposed to five or ten potential sources of infection.

Keep in mind that it is current practice to separate the platelets from a single unit of donated blood. However, the amount of useful platelets that can be harvested from a single unit of blood is relatively small. When one needs a platelet transfusion, six or eight or even ten units of blood are frequently required to yield the necessary amount of useful platelets. This means that one is exposed to six or eight or even ten potentially infected donors.

In many cases of surgery, the exposure from platelet administration is even greater than from red cell or plasma transfusion. A patient undergoing heart surgery, for example, might receive five units of red cells, four units of plasma, and ten packs of platelets, thus risking exposure to a total of 19 different donors. As will be shown, this massive number of donors can be reduced to a tiny fraction using the single-donor or "monodonor" method.

One of the special problems of receiving platelets from multiple donors is that patients quickly develop antibodies to various donor platelets. It then becomes increasingly difficult to give additional platelet transfusions because the platelets are rapidly destroyed. Platelet antibodies can form rapidly; they may develop within a few days. One of the ways of preventing the development of platelet antibodies is to obtain as many as six or eight platelet packs from a single healthy donor. This can be accomplished through the technique of plateletpheresis—a variant of plasmapheresis—wherein blood is removed from a donor and cycled through a continuously pumping machine that separates the platelets out while simultaneously returning the rest of the blood, minus the platelets, to the patient. Using plateletpheresis, one is able to skim off a large amount of platelets without causing harm to the body.

It may seem surprising, but in a healthy donor, the equivalent of six to eight platelet packs can be safely removed and still leave enough healthy platelets to provide a good margin of safety. Healthy donors are able to replenish most missing platelets within five to ten days. The body has a significant reserve and, in contrast to lost blood, is able to replace lost platelets very rapidly.

In certain conditions such as leukemias and lymphomas, however, patients need repeated platelet transfusions. However, it is absolutely essential that the platelet donations come from a single donor; otherwise the recipient becomes so sensitized that he destroys any platelets he receives and further transfusion becomes impossible.

Given the present, known danger of platelet transfusions, it is difficult to justify giving an individual platelets from six or eight different donors when it is possible to obtain the same number of platelets from a single donor. Blood bankers may argue that this will result in some wasting of platelets from individual donors. While this is true, cost considerations should not take precedence over safety concerns. It is far safer to use monodonors instead of multiple donors for platelet transfusions, since the same amount of platelets can be obtained from a single donor, with a manifold reduction in risk. In the age of AIDS, the fewer donors one is exposed to, the better are one's chances of avoiding infection; one gains the additional advantage of not developing antibodies to numerous donors.

As mentioned earlier, platelets are difficult to freeze. At the present time, the technology for freezing platelets is only moderately successful and a significant number cannot be recovered intact. The solution has been to have human donors available on short notice for platelet transfusion emergencies. However, a combination of frozen and fresh monodonor (single-donor) platelets can be used to avoid multiple exposure. The blood bank of the future will therefore use monodoors as the standard form of platelet replacement instead of the current practice of one donor per transfusion, which considerably magnifies the risk. When all the platelets come from a single preselected donor, the risk of infection or transfusion reaction is significantly reduced, if not eliminated.

Multiple donor platelet transfusions should be used as a backup when there are inadequate supplies of monodonors. There is a real need for individuals who are willing to serve as platelet donors.

An additional problem with platelets arises from their very short life span of 6 to 7 days. Many blood banking facilities are unable to complete their blood tests in less than 72 hours and under these circumstances, platelets are already 3 days old when used for transfusion. When platelets are frozen, their aging is stopped. But until frozen platelets can be fully and effectively utilized, a monodonor system coupled with a 24-hour laboratory turnaround can provide useable platelets from a single donor. To alleviate this problem now, the FDA permits tests performed on the donor up to 30 days earlier to be applied to the platelets. However, in this case, no direct tests are carried out on the platelets themselves.

REDUCING DONOR EXPOSURE

Consider a patient who undergoes either a coronary bypass or extensive abdominal surgery and has lost six pints of blood out of a total volume of nine—in other words, someone who has lost two-thirds of his blood supply, a loss incompatible with life unless there is some replacement.

Obviously such a patient would be receiving transfusions during the course of his surgery—or at least volume replacement with salt water; otherwise he would not be able to survive. Typically, such a patient might wind up after surgery with as much as 90 or 95 percent of his platelets lost or used up. He would lose even more platelets than red cells or plasma because, in addition to the platelets lost in the blood, the system uses up its platelets in an attempt to stem bleeding within the body.

Typically a patient in the initial stages of major surgery would be replaced with red cells and plasma but not platelets. Indeed, there would be no platelets given at all until the body's platelet count dropped to a drastically low level. Only if a patient receives red cells and plasma from very fresh whole blood will effective platelets still be present. However, this is almost never the case, since the oldest blood in a blood bank is always used first to prevent stores from outdating.

Today the patient who lost 6 pints of blood might be replaced with four units of red cells, four units of plasma and eight units of platelets for a total donor exposure of 16.* To understand this concept, one

*This would be a typical example of doctors undertransfusing their patients for blood loss. Obviously to be missing two pints of blood after undergoing extensive surgery is far from ideal.

should examine Table 3, which is based on a six-pint blood loss with only partial replacement of the lost blood. It illustrates variances in donor exposure as a function of the number of units of blood stored by an individual. To use this table, one should begin by looking at line I and read across: when zero units of blood are stored, the total donor exposure is 16 separate donors. Line II shows the drastic reduction in donor exposure—from 16 donors to 3—when only a single unit of blood is stored by an individual. This table should be examined closely (and with some patience) to grasp the remarkable reduction in donor exposure that is possible with only modest amounts of blood storage.

Table 4 shows a six-pint blood loss with complete replacement. The concept of total blood replacement, which is ideal for the patient, is possible with only limited donor exposure when one uses the modern "monodonor" or unidonor system. In this case, the patient could receive full replacement for her lost six pints of blood—six units of red cells, six units of plasma, and eight packs of platelets—and still be exposed to only a single donor instead of 20, providing she has stored just three pints of her own blood. In addition, after transfusion, this patient would have a full supply of blood instead of being depleted and anemic.

Currently, a patient who received full replacement for his lost six pints of blood would require six red cell donors, six plasma donors, and eight platelet donors, and would therefore be exposed to a total of 20 donors—or 20 potential sources of infection (Table 4, line I). If this same patient had the foresight to store three units of his own blood and three from a matching friend or family member, he could then receive three units of his own red cells and plasma; he could also receive an additional three units of red cells and plasma from his friend or relative; furthermore, that single friend or relative could be utilized on an emergency basis to provide the needed platelets. The patient in this example would therefore be exposed to a single known donor instead of 20 unknown donors and still receive the same amount of blood (Table 4, line IV). In addition, he would reap the benefit of having a fully normal supply of blood.

Alternatively, an individual might store only two units of blood and have family members or friends store another two units each (Table 4, line III) Under these circumstances, the patient would receive two units of her own red cells and 2 units of her own plasma; then two units of red cells and two of plasma from a relative; then another two units of red cells and two of plasma from another friend or

Table 3   Donor Exposure from Partial Replacement of 6-Pint Blood Loss

	A Number of Units Stored	B Red Cell Donors	C Plasma Donors	D Platelet Donors	E Total Donors
I	0	4	4	8	16
II	1	3	0	0	3
III	2	1	0	0	1
IV	3	1	0	0	1

Table 3 shows the number of donors to whom a patient with a massive six-pint blood loss would be exposed if he received partial replacement—a typical situation today. In this case, two pints would be replaced with water, leaving four units of red cells, four units of plasma and eight platelet units to be replaced. When no blood is stored (I-A) a patient is exposed to 16 donors (I-E). By contrast, when three units are stored (IV-A), a patient is exposed to only one donor (IV-E). Note that with a three-unit storage system, he could be given full replacement with no extra risk. As can be seen from both tables, family members do not have to store huge quantities of blood to benefit from a major reduction in risk.

Table 4   Donor Exposure from Full Replacement of 6-Pint Blood Loss

	A Number of Units Stored	B Red Cell Donors	C Plasma Donors	D Platelet Donors	E Total Donors
I	0	6	6	8	20
II	1	5	0	0	5
III	2	2	0	0	2
IV	3	1	0	0	1

Table 4 shows the number of donors to whom a patient with a massive six-pint blood loss would be exposed if she received full blood replacement. Column A indicates the number of units stored by participating family members. When no blood is stored (I-A), a patient is exposed to 20 different donors (I-E) in order to get back her six missing units. By contrast, when three units of blood are stored by each member (IV-A), a patient is exposed to only 1 donor (IV-E), in addition to receiving her own three units. Note the dramatic drop from 20 donors (I-E) to 5 donors (II-E) when even only a single unit is stored by each family member.

relative. Again, one of these two donors would then serve as the platelet monodonor.

Under these circumstances, one is exposed to 2 known donors instead of 20 anonymous donors. In addition, these 2 donors have had their blood tested, frozen, stored, and retested, so it is almost certain they do not have AIDS or hepatitis—in contrast to the 20 screened but anonymous donors who have not been retested for AIDS or hepatitis. Even if the known and selected donors were no safer than anonymous donors, the reduction from 20 to 2 is a vast improvement. If the patient is only partially replaced, which would be the more standard method (see Table 3, line III) he would actually require only a single donor despite this very large, six-pint loss of blood.

Consider further an individual who is to have full replacement of a six-pint blood loss and has stored only a single unit of blood for herself, while five of her relatives have stored one unit each (Table 4, line II). Under these conditions, the patient would receive one unit of her own red cells and one unit of her own plasma, in addition to five more units of red cells and the five units of plasma from five different relatives. Any one of these five relatives could be the potential platelet monodonor. Under these circumstances, where only a single unit of blood was stored by the patient, she will be exposed to 5 known, retested donors instead of 20 anonymous donors for full blood replacement. If only partial replacement is given (see Table 3, line II), then she would be exposed to 3 donors instead of 16.

Clearly, even the storage of a single unit of blood by family and friends markedly reduces the risk from a blood transfusion. Keep in mind that we have deliberately used an extreme example in which an individual loses six pints of blood or more than half the blood in her body. In a more typical situation, where one might lose three or four pints of blood, one would not need to be exposed to any outside donors at all if one had stored one or two units of blood in advance.

Since blood types are inherited, it is not difficult to organize a blood program with relatives that provides significant protection from the risks of transfusion. It is also possible to keep costs low by having one or two individuals with the most common blood type store three or four units of blood which can be used by most other members of the family. Even shared blood storage between compatible friends markedly reduces the risk.

Additional steps could be taken by the blood banks themselves to reduce donor exposure. Their current practice is to separate a unit of whole blood into red cells, plasma, and platelets and transfuse each component into a separate patient. Instead, they should ensure that each patient receives red cells, plasma, and platelets from the same donor wherever possible. Such a change would create some extra bookkeeping for blood banks, but given the high risk of infection today, it is unacceptable not to make every attempt to lower donor exposure.

Similar precautions should be taken with respect to infants. Premature infants frequently receive tiny transfusions called "quadpacks." In these situations, a regular-sized component of red cells might be broken up into four or five subcomponents, because infants may only need a small amount of blood at one time. Blood banks will usually deliver all the components intact to a hospital, but many hospitals will then split up the packs and make no attempt to transfuse the infant with blood components from the same donor.

In a case decided by the San Francisco Superior Court, a premature infant boy was transfused with blood from 18 different donors, 1 of whom gave him AIDS. Yet only 6 donors could have sufficed to meet the child's needs if basic steps had been taken to keep the various blood packs intact. In this particular case the family attempted to donate blood for the newborn baby but was turned down by the blood bank and the hospital. The family sued and lost, in a case typifying the freedom from liability granted to the blood industry.[9] Ironically, had the family been permitted to donate its own blood and had certain other steps been taken, all of the infant's blood needs could have been supplied from only four family members. In addition, by permitting the family to donate, the hospital and blood bank would have helped to alleviate the blood shortage rather than aggravating it.

When it comes to limiting donor exposure—and maximizing the transfusion recipient's safety—no effort should be spared. In the blood bank of the future, such basic precautions will be permanent features of a safe and optimum blood supply system.

EXPERIMENTAL CONCEPTS

Many people feel unconcerned about problems in the blood supply because they believe that medical science is so advanced today that it is only a matter of time before artificial blood or some other new remedy is found. While there is much ongoing research in hematology and immunology—and many short-lived claims about the discovery of a new elixir—nevertheless, as of today there is no likely substitute for human blood nor any safe method to cleanse blood of all its contaminants. Following is a brief look at the most talked-about, experimental concepts.

Artificial Blood

The idea of man-made blood has attracted doctors and scientists for over 25 years. Periodically, reports have surfaced of a breakthrough or near breakthrough in the search for an infection-free, immunologically neutral alternative to normal blood transfusions. Unfortunately, no such blood substitute has yet been developed.

The liquid perfluorocarbon emulsions that were hailed in the 1970s as blood substitutes have not lived up to their promise.[10] This synthetic blood was made from fluorocarbons, an oxygen-carrying substance that is chemically similar to synthetic oils and can be manufactured in near-perfect sterility. But fluorocarbons have proven unable to carry enough oxygen to compensate for emergency blood losses or shock. They normally carry about 10 percent of oxygen for total volume, whereas 40 to 50 percent is required. Another problem has been that these blood substitutes can trigger severe transfusion reactions.

A few years ago, Japanese scientists developed a new blood substitute, Fluosol-DA, which they claimed was safer and more effective than previous fluorocarbons. However, results from a randomized trial in California showed that there was almost no difference between patients who received the emulsion and those who did not. As a result the FDA has restricted use of this fluorocarbon to Jehovah's Witnesses, since they refuse any transfusion with human blood.[11]

A slightly more promising type of artificial blood has been made out of discarded hemoglobin. The naked hemoglobin molecules are removed from red cells and linked into long chains that carry oxygen through the blood system. Some studies have shown that animals can survive with nothing but this chemically modified hemoglobin in their system. This kind of artificial blood has served as a temporary palliative in experimental studies. But preliminary findings suggest that, at best, it is good for only a few days. In addition, artificial hemoglobin is highly toxic to the kidneys. Therefore this experimental, artificial blood has no practical application in humans at the present time.

Despite continuing research, there is no serious blood substitute on the scientific horizon today. No one is even close to making an artificial red cell, while hemoglobin outside of a red cell remains highly toxic and dangerous. Hence, today artificial blood is not a realistic alternative to human blood for transfusions.

Blood Cleansing

One solution for dealing with the host of infectious agents transmitted by blood is to find a safe method of cleansing or sterilizing blood of its viral contaminants. Plasma products such as Factor VIII are presently treated by complex heating techniques to deactivate viruses. In the past, other methods that were thought to be effective have proven disastrous. The tragedy of 10,000 hemophiliacs—half the nation's hemophiliac population—who were infected with AIDS from Factor VIII is a chilling example of the consequences of inadequate treatment of blood. Present techniques to deactivate viruses in plasma products are believed to be more effective.

Whole blood and blood components have generally proven even more resistant to antiviral agents. It is difficult to kill off infectious agents in the blood without damaging the integrity and full functional capability of the blood elements. Recent efforts to deactivate blood-borne viruses have concentrated on the use of laser beams and chemicals. By adding certain dyes and using special light beams it may be possible to kill off some viruses. The photodynamic approach offers the chance to select viral targets without resorting to potent toxic agents.

Preliminary results from Baylor University in Texas suggest that enveloped viruses are more susceptible to photodynamic attack—dye and light exposure—than naked viruses.[12] This finding could have potential relevance to HIV, which has a viral envelope. However, HIV is found *inside* T lymphocytes and monocytes, which means that just cleaning the blood itself will not kill the virus inside the cells. The only way to do so may be to kill the cells themselves. It would not appear that intracellular viruses are as susceptible to attack with the dye as are the free viruses. Another problem remaining to be overcome is removal of the dye that combines with the blood. To date, this has not been effectively dealt with.

Further tests and studies are necessary to investigate these possibilities. As of today, there is still no safe, sure method for cleansing and sterilizing blood of its contaminants in such a way that blood itself is not destroyed or rendered unsafe for transfusion.

Bone-Marrow Stimulator

A new and promising development has been the synthesis of a genetically engineered human protein called erythropoietin, which stimulates bone marrow to produce red blood cells. By increasing blood production, this drug can be used to increase the amount of blood donated prior to surgery and to speed recovery of blood lost during surgery.

In contrast to blood cleansing and artificial blood, manufactured erythropoietin is a genuine advance that will help—but not eliminate—the blood transfusion problem. It will definitely decrease the need for blood in some cases, such as kidney disease. Erythropoietin is a hormone produced naturally by the kidney, but many people whose health is compromised have a deficiency in erythropoietin and a suppressed bone marrow. The genetically engineered replica of the natural hormone will stimulate the marrow to make blood cells and help speed up the blood-making capabilities of the human body. In June 1989 it won preliminary approval for treatment of a severe anemia that afflicts many AIDS patients.[13]

While useful, this drug, which has since been approved by the FDA,[14] will nevertheless have only limited value. It may shorten the time necessary to make up a pint of blood from four to two weeks—a significant improvement. But it will not provide an adequate supply of blood. While erythropoietin will no doubt prove helpful in cases of chronic blood loss, it will have little effect where there is sudden loss and a need for larger amounts of blood, such as one to two pints required within a one- or two-day period. In such cases, a blood transfusion is required.

PERSONAL RESPONSIBILITY

The foregoing chapters have demonstrated the myriad risks associated with blood transfusions today and outlined alternative steps that can be taken to provide greater safety for blood recipients. However, until the government and the blood banking establishment admit to the current danger in the blood supply and take major corrective action, it is up to each of us to look after his or her own blood needs.

The blood banking establishment has many powerful reasons for opposing any change that might threaten its historic monopoly; but the public has also allowed itself to be misled. The time has come when ignorance about basic transfusion policies can no longer be justified. As citizens we must seek to inform and involve ourselves individually so that we can make the best practical decisions for our own blood needs and those of our families. In the absence of a strong public response, individual action is the only sane course for responsible citizens to take.

One should select a blood storage facility with the same care one would use in selecting a surgeon. Shop around and carefully research the background and capability of any group or company offering to store blood. To date, at least 19 companies have entered and left the blood storage business, many of them having gone bankrupt. Most were undercapitalized and could not generate enough interest from the public before their financing ran out. The technical and financial assets, as well as the commitment, of the blood bank facility you choose should be carefully checked. Avoid such enticements as contracts that offer the right to store multiple units of blood for one initial, large, fixed fee. Organizations offering this kind of deal may be out of business by the time you are ready to store your second or third unit. A reputable organization that expects to stay in business should be willing to accept a partial fee for only a single unit of blood stored for a few months. Remember, too, that a good facility can be situated at a considerable distance and still get blood to you if proper transportational logistics have been worked out.

Any blood bank that ships blood across state lines—most autologous banks offer this service—must be licensed by the Food and Drug Administration. The rules and regulations governing these frozen banks are the same as the rules that govern voluntary blood facilities. The banks are inspected at least once a year and must meet all FDA criteria, as well as local standards. When selecting a personal blood storage facility, you should request to see a copy of the blood bank's FDA license. If there is any doubt, you can call the FDA directly and verify that the bank is licensed. You should also ask the blood bank for a reference list of hospitals that have accepted and used its blood. Making certain that your blood bank is professionally recognized by your hospital and physician will ensure that no last-minute snags develop. Get a list of clients as well, and verify that their stored blood was, in fact, sent to the hospital and used effectively.

Some doctors and hospitals are reluctant to cooperate because using frozen autologous blood requires extra effort and time on their part, for which they may receive no additional compensation. You must remember to be assertive about your right to have safe blood available. If you pick your own doctor, make sure he or she understands your wishes concerning a blood transfusion and agrees to cooperate in advance.

Another major form of accreditation to check is that of the American Association of Blood Banks. While we have made some critical remarks about the AABB's lack of aggressiveness in upgrading standards, it is nevertheless the premier accrediting organization in the United States for quality control in blood banking. A good blood bank should at least be able to meet all AABB standards. The AABB provides accreditation and certification, which can be checked through their office in Arlington, Va.

Investigate your frozen blood bank as thoroughly as you wish, but once you have found a reputable firm, you should act quickly. Do not neglect to store your own blood *before* you ever need it. If you are unable to freeze your own blood, the next best thing is to designate the donor whose blood you wish to receive and have him or her store for you. Some people argue that designated donors are no safer than anonymous donors from the general supply. They fear that relatives and close friends will feel pressured to donate in an emergency and might not divulge all the details of their private lives. Yet many blood drives today, particularly at corporations and large institutions, similarly involve a high degree of coercion. When the blood drive director is one's own boss or supervisor, pressure to donate may be just as intense, if not more so, than from a relative. In a well-known case documented by the CDC,[15] a donor implicated in a transfusion-associated AIDS case turned out to be the chairman of his company's blood drive. Though he was a homosexual—a member of a known high-risk blood category asked not to donate—he nevertheless felt pressured to donate.

Indeed, designated donors may be safer than anonymous donors in several ways. First, simply matching platelets, plasma, and red cells from one designated donor—instead of the three now used for each component—minimizes exposure to potential sources of infection. Second, if the designated donor is a blood relative, the chances of a good match between the 600 or more blood subtypes are much improved, and the risk of a transfusion reaction correspondingly reduced. A recent minor concern has been that blood donations between close relatives might result in a rare graft-verus-host reaction due to white cells from the donor. This situation is extremely rare. More significantly, when frozen blood is thawed and separated, the white cells are washed out along with the antifreeze agent used to protect the red cells, markedly reducing the rare possibility of graft versus host reaction.* Third, it has recently been shown that platelets obtained from a donor of the same blood type have significantly better survival within the bloodstream than those from unmatched blood donors. Fourth, several studies have shown that simple selection based on sex—female donors are safer than males[16]—would be advisable. Fifth, although it is hard to quantify, there is also psychological benefit of knowing that one is receiving blood from a relative or friend. According to some, that assurance may actually aid recuperation.[17] Finally, under a frozen blood system, designated donors would be retested along with all others after a suitable interval for any sign of AIDS or hepatitis. Obviously donors who have been tested twice, six months or more apart, are markedly safer than anonymous donors from the general blood supply who have been tested only once. Clearly, the monodonor and family stored blood program provides for the basic possibility of having one's own safe blood available when it is needed and for the possibility of markedly reducing donor exposure in comparison to the present system.

CONCLUSION

The American public has been misled by a series of false assurances concerning the safety of the nation's blood supply. The reason that these misrepresentations have not resulted in disastrous legal judgments against the organizations making them has been the extraordinary legislative immunity that has long protected the blood banking establishment from liability. The recent spate of lawsuits challenging this immunity may have the beneficial effect of forcing honest disclosure about the real risks of blood transfusions.

Major blood organizations have long benefited from the semantic distinction between selling a service and selling a product. This legal nicety should not protect them from the consequences of making false assurances about the safety of a service directly affecting the 4 million Americans who require a blood transfusion each year. Just as a cardiac surgeon is legally liable if he falsely claims that the risk of a

---

*In fresh directed or designated donations between close relatives, it might be useful to uniformly wash out the white cells prior to transfusion. Other scientists have suggested simple short-term radiation treatment to the blood prior to transfusion to eliminate this rare possibility.

fatal outcome from heart surgery is one in a million, blood banking organizations should also be liable, and responsible, for what they say and do. Misleading statements about the safety of the nation's blood supply are particularly damaging because they lull the public into a false sense of security and prevent individuals from seeking other available options to provide safer blood for themselves and their families.

The technological and logistical possibilities for a safe and adequate blood supply exist today. These posibilities center on the use of frozen autologous blood, supplemented by blood from a limited, personally selected donor pool. In addition, all blood banks should immediately implement the administrative changes that are necessary to reduce multiple donor exposure to an absolute minimum.

The expected reduction of infection from preventable hepatitis alone would be in excess of 90 percent—preventing this disease in over 200,000 Americans each year who contract it from a blood transfusion. It would also save thousands of hepatitis victims who die every year from cirrhosis. The 90 percent reduction will result from the use of one's own blood and the introduction of the monodonor concept, whereby exposure to multiple donors is reduced to an absolute minimum. It is important to remember that while a new test for one form of hepatitis non-A, non-B,—the so-called "hepatitis C"—will lower the risk of hepatitis in the blood supply, there will still be many thousands of cases, and many other forms of hepatitis non-A, non-B, that will not be detected by this test. In addition, new blood-borne diseases such as Chagas' and Lyme disease are now recognized as being potentially transmissible via a blood transfusion—a risk that is virtually eliminated when one stores one's own blood.

The use of a frozen blood system will also eliminate over 95 percent of the hundreds, possibly thousands, of new cases of transfusion-AIDS that still occur each year. As previously demonstrated, the incidence of AIDS transmitted through transfusions is substantially higher than the public perceives. The use of frozen blood should significantly reduce AIDS from the blood supply—as it has already reduced AIDS from sperm used in artificial insemination donations.

A nationwide frozen autologous blood program in conjunction with a limited donor-directed program will thus more than pay for itself by saving lives and preventing the hundreds of new cases of transfusion-AIDS, and the thousands of new cases of transfusion-hepatitis, every year. For those using their own blood, it will also provide perfectly matched blood and almost completely eliminate the risks of transfusion reaction. The use of frozen autologous blood, coupled with a monodonor system where additional blood is needed, will also significantly reduce the unacknowledged complications resulting from undertransfusion of severely ill patients. American public health will be vastly improved and American citizens provided with essential medical safeguards that they now lack.

Another major advantage will be the virtual elimination of the continuing crisis of blood shortages. In effect, we are operating blood banks in the 1990s with some of the methodologies of the 1940s. No nation with a modern health system should function with a zero-to-two-day blood supply. The autologous and designated blood programs we have described will go far toward eliminating this problem.

Human blood is not only life's most precious fluid; it is also our most private, intimate substance, unique to each individual. None of us should be forced to accept foreign blood from a total stranger—particularly when it has a well-documented risk of infection. The only safe blood is your own, and the only sure way to have your own blood available when you need it is to store it well in advance of any anticipated need.

The present blood banking system has been responsible for saving thousands of lives; yet while its leading organizations include many dedicated and able professionals, these organizations did not take steps that might have prevented thousands of avoidable deaths and many thousands of unnecessary and avoidable complications. The unqualified trust that we have traditionally placed in this system can no longer be justified. We cannot afford to think otherwise. But we *can* act to change and improve it. When it comes to blood banking, the public benefit can best be served in a system that respects the right of the individual to take an active role in his or her own health care.

Existing organizations have played and should continue to play an important and major role in providing the nation's blood supply. It is essential that people donate blood for general use, and it is also important that the number of people who donate blood should be vastly expanded. At the same time, the potential exists for a major new means of supplying safe blood by way of a system in which individuals will take greater responsibility for their own blood needs and those of their families. Considering the known risks of transfusion today—and the unknown risks of tomorrow—it is imperative that we move forward to implement this new plan for safe blood. It should increase our satisfaction to know that while protecting our own health, each of us will also contribute to the improved health and well-being of the community at large.

Notes

CHAPTER 1
A Dangerous Misunderstanding

1. New York Blood Center, Public Information Department, "Some Facts about Blood Transfusions," 1988.

2. See, for example, Ross Eckert, "Blood, Money and Monopoly," in *Securing a Safer Blood Supply: Two Views* (Washington, D.C.: American Enterprise Institute, 1985), p. 3.

3. Gary L. Davis et al., "Treatment of Chronic Hepatitis C with Recombinant Interferon Alfa," *New England Journal of Medicine* 321 (November 1989):1501–5. Davis reports: "Hepatitis C (non-A, non-B) is a common disease that accounts for more than 90% of cases of hepatitis that develop after transfusion. Despite improvement in the quality of the blood donor pool and the recent implementation of testing of donated blood, the current estimated incidence of acute infections among persons receiving transfusion is 5 to 10 percent." The article estimates that there are 150,000 new cases of hepatitis non-A, non-B each year in people who receive a transfusion. This figure is based on 3 million transfusion recipients annually, whereas there are approximately 4 million blood recipients each year. (See Ross Eckert, "Statement on Blood Safety," in *Report of the Presidential Commission on the Human Immunodeficiency Virus Epidemic,* No. 0-214-701 [Washington, D.C.: U.S. Governmental Printing Office, 1988], p. 1.) The 150,000 figure is also based on the lower 5 percent estimate. Using the official Red Cross figure of 4 million transfusion recipients a year, one must assume that there are anywhere between 200,000 and 400,000 people annually who develop hepatitis non-A, non-B from a blood transfusion. This number does not

181

even take into account those who develop hepatitis B. See also J. H. Alter, "Transfusion-Associated non-A, non-B Hepatitis: The First Decade," in A. J. Zuckerman, ed., *Viral Hepatitis and Liver Disease* (New York: Alan R. Liss, 1988), pp. 537–42. The new hepatitis C test may eliminate as many as 50 percent of these transfusion-hepatitis cases, which would still leave between 100,000 and 200,000 new cases each year.

4. J. D. Kalbfleisch and J. F. Lawless, "Estimating the Incubation Time Distribution and Expected Number of Cases of Transfusion-Associated Acquired Immune Deficiency Syndrome," *Transfusion* 29 (October 1989): 672–76. These researchers estimate that there will be between 14,300 and 15,000 eventual cases of AIDS—in the age group 13 to 69—attributable to infection by blood transfusion prior to June 1985. This figure is an upward revision of the previous CDC figure of 12,000. See Centers for Disease Control, Atlanta, "Human Immunodeficiency Virus Infection in Transfusion Recipients and Their Family Members," *Morbidity and Mortality Weekly Report* 36 (1987):137–40.

5. Gilbert C. White II et al., "Use of Recombinant Antihemophilic Factor in the Treatment of Two Patients with Classic Hemophilia," *New England Journal of Medicine* 320 (January 1989):166–72. See also R. C. Gallo et al., "Frequent Detection and Isolation of Cytopathic Retroviruses (HTLV-III) from patients with AIDS and at Risk for AIDS," *Science* 224 (1984):500–503, and J. J. Goedert et al., "Antibodies Reactive with Human T Cell Leukemia Viruses in the Serum of Hemophiliacs Receiving Factor VIII Concentrate," *Blood* 65 (1985):472–75. Other estimates have placed the number of hemophiliacs infected with AIDS as a result of contaminated clotting factor at 12,000. See Gilbert Gaul, "America: OPEC of Global Plasma Industry," *Philadelphia Inquirer,* September 26, 1989.

6. This figure is derived partly from the CDC estimate that the risk of AIDS per transfusion unit is 1 in 40,000. See J. W. Ward et al., "Transmission of Human Immunodeficiency Virus (HIV) Infection by Blood Transfusion Screened as Negative for HIV Antibody," *New England Journal of Medicine* 318 (February 1988): 473–78, as well as subsequent quotes by Dr. Ward in Robert Steinbrook's "Transfusion AIDS risk scaled back," *Los Angeles Times,* October 5, 1989, p. 38. It is derived also from the Red Cross estimate that the average transfusion comprises 5.4 units. See Cummings et al., "Exposure of Patients," *New England Journal of Medicine* 321 (October 1989): 941. Dividing 40,000 by 5.4, we arrive at 7,400, which means that the average risk of contracting AIDS for each patient who receives a blood transfusion may be 1 in 7,400.

7. Food and Drug Administration memorandum, "Recommendations for Changeover from Use of Fresh Immunizing Red Blood Cells to Use of Frozen Immunizing Red Blood Cells Stored a Minimum of Six Months Prior to Use," *Plasmapheresis,* November 1988, p. 264.

8. David T. Imagawa et al., "Human Immunodeficiency Virus Type 1 Infection in Homosexual Men Who Remain Seronegative for Prolonged Periods," *New England Journal of Medicine* 320 (June 1989): 1458–62.

9. FDA and CDC, "Risks of Transmitting AIDS via Donor Organs, Tissue and Sperm Used in Artificial Insemination," *Morbidity and Mortality Weekly Report* 37 (February 5, 1988): 1, as reported in the *American Association of Tissue Banks Newsletter* 11 (1988): 1.

10. With reference to artificial insemination, it should be noted that the FDA stopped short of setting up mandatory screening procedures, issuing voluntary guidelines only—a move for which they have been sharply criticized by the Congressional Office of Technology Assessment. Senator Albert Gore called this half-measure "deeply troubling" and went on to say: "The FDA, by failing to set policy, is endangering the lives of these (172,000) women and the health of their offspring." See Jeff Nesmith, "Many Sperm Donors Aren't Screened for Diseases," *Atlanta Journal and Constitution*, April 3, 1988, p. 12.

11. *Report of Presidential Commission*, p. 78. The report lists this special relationship between the FDA and the blood banking establishment as an "Obstacle to Progress."

12. This figure was cited by Thomas M. Asher in a report entitled "Blood— A Hazardous Monopoly," delivered to the Presidential Commission on the HIV Epidemic, May 9, 1988 (p. 2).

13. Ibid.

14. The American Red Cross annual report for the year ending June 1987 lists total revenues for the Blood Services at $521,885,000 (p. 23). The figure for 1989 is expected to be higher. For a vivid sense of the profits involved, see also Andrea Rock, "Inside the Billion-Dollar Business of Blood," *Money*, March 1986, p. 158ff.

15. The American Red Cross annual report for the year ending June 1987 shows that 76% of its total revenues came from "Blood Services Processing" (p. 30). However, in testimony before Congress in June 1987, Dr. Lewellys Barker, senior vice president of the American Red Cross, disagreed with this number when confronted by Chairman Pickle of the Subcommittee on Oversight: "Mr. Chairman, first I would slightly modify this figure. Our blood services revenues account for roughly 60 per cent of total Red Cross revenue and roughly 40 per cent comes from philanthropy, endowment income and other sources." Unrelated Business Income Tax (UBIT) Hearings before the Subcommittee on Oversight, House Committee on Ways and Means, One Hundredth Congress, First Session, Part 2 of 3. June 26 and 29, 1987, p. 1086.

16. Based on Andrea Rock's finding that "Sales of plasma derivatives now account for about 15% of the Blood Services' annual revenues" in her article "Billion-Dollar Business," p. 160.

17. These advantages, mentioned in several sources, were neatly summarized by Thomas Asher in testimony before the Subcommittee on Oversight Investigating Unrelated Business Income Tax, June 26, 1986, p. 1085.

18. UBIT Hearings, p. 2. In appointing the subcommittee, Dan Rostenkowski, chairman of the House Ways and Means Committee, noted: "In recent years, exempt organizations have become more aggressive in undertaking commercial or enterpreneurial activities. For-profit businesses have complained that tax-exempt organizations are provided an unfair competitive advantage under present tax law. Indeed this issue of unfair competition now has reached national prominence as demonstrated by the designation of this issue as a priority item in the recent national White House Conference on Small Business."

19. UBIT Hearings, p. 1080.

20. Richard Titmuss, *The Gift Relationship: From Human Blood to Social Policy* (New York: Vintage Books, 1972).

21. Eckert, "Blood, Money and Monopoly," p. 77.

22. There is now a broad consensus concerning this failure. See, among others, Edgar Engleman, "AIDS and the Blood Supply," *Report of Presidential Commission;* Rock, "Billion-Dollar Business"; Eckert, "Blood, Money and Monopoly"; and Randy Shilts, *And the Band Played On: People, Politics and the AIDS Epidemic* (New York: St. Martin's Press, 1987). The Presidential Commission on the HIV Epidemic, despite its politically sensitive position, also found that the blood banking industry was "unnecessarily slow" in its initial reaction to the threat of AIDS contamination in the blood supply. *Report of Presidential Commission.*

23. Sandra Blakeslee, "Blood Banks Facing Hundreds of AIDS Suits," *New York Times,* April 27, 1989.

24. Engleman, "AIDS and the Blood Supply," p. 10.

25. Joan Ferran, "Ensuring the Gift of Life," *Central Florida,* December 1985. Ferran reviews the well-publicized case of Richard Studer and his son which began in the summer of 1983.

26. The case involving St. Joseph's Hospital is now before the Superior Court of New Jersey. As recently as April of 1989, the director of a major hospital in New York refused to permit stored, frozen blood from a seriously ill patient's wife and son to be given to that patient. Instead, the patient was forced to choose between dying from lack of blood or accepting anonymous blood from the general supply.

27. The case of O'Rourke v. Irwin Memorial Blood Bank, Children's Hospital of San Francisco, was decided in favor of the blood bank.

28. Rock, "Billion-Dollar Business," p. 162 ff.; Eckert, "AIDS and the Blood Bankers," pp. 18–19.

29. Eckert, "AIDS and the Blood Bankers," *Regulation,* September/October 1986, p. 18.

30. Rock, "Billion-Dollar Business," pp. 165–66; Engleman, "AIDS and the Blood Supply," pp. 3–6.

31. Rock, "Billion-Dollar Business," pp. 163, 167.

32. See notes 4 and 5.

33. Engleman, "AIDS and the Blood Supply," p. 9.

34. Ibid., p. 10.

35. There does exist a potentially direct test for the AIDS virus in the blood, a test that uses DNA amplification techniques. However, at the present time, this test is too difficult and too expensive to perform routinely.

36. Imagawa, "Human Immunodeficiency Virus."

37. Gina Kolata, "AIDS Virus Found to Hide in Cells, Eluding Detection by Normal Tests," *New York Times,* June 5, 1988, p. 1.

38. Randolph Wykoff and Neal Halsey, "The Effectiveness of Voluntary Self-Exclusion on Blood Donation Practices of Individuals at High Risk for AIDS," *Journal of the American Medical Association* 256 (1986): 1292–93. See also S. F. Leitman et al., "Clinical Implications of Positive Tests for Antibodies to Human Immunodeficiency Virus Type 1 in Asymptomatic Blood Donors," *New England Journal of Medicine* 321 (October 1989): 917–24.

39. See, for example, L. Montagnier and S. Wain-Hobson, "The AIDS Virus: Structure and Variation," in J. C. Petricciani et al., *AIDS: The Safety of Blood and Blood Products* (New York: Wiley, 1987), p. 8. In the World Health Organization conference recorded here Dr. B. Habibi points out that there are "more than 7 isolates from different parts of the world" and that this "variation may evolve in the same patient over time."

Dr. Habibi goes on to raise a very difficult question: " 'So with this background the point I would like to raise is that the tremendous amount of effort and cost devoted to large-scale screening of blood donors can hardly be justified if the antigenic material in our test kit does not actually cover the whole range of viruses for the present time and future mutants. I would like to know if others share this same anxiety about this potential difficulty faced by blood transfusion facilities.' (No response)"

40. Ross Eckert, "Statement on Blood Supply," p. 3: "This is a staggering statistic. Assuming transfusion cirrhosis is fatal, losing 4000 people per year is roughly like losing the passengers on one fully-loaded DC-10 every month." Even this figure may be low, since Eckert accepts the blood industry's unsubstantiated claims that it has reduced the general risk of hepatitis to 5 percent. See Chapter 5 for a more realistic, and chilling, assessment.

41. Leonard Sloane, "Increasingly, Blood Recipients Are Getting Their Own Blood," *New York Times*, November 10, 1988. Confirmed in conversation with the American Association of Blood Banks, December 1988.

42. The American Red Cross, *Blood Services Annual Report 1986–1987* (Washington, D.C.: ARC, 1988), p. 4, states: "The safest blood for any patient is his or her own. However, for various reasons, only 10% of those who need it may be able to give blood for themselves." The real figure may be closer to 5 percent—see Chapter 8.

43. National Institutes of Health, "Consensus Conference," *Journal of the American Medical Association* 260, no. 18 (November 11, 1988).

44. The New York Blood Center publication "Some Facts About Blood Donation" places the figure at 3 percent for the New York area.

45. Marianne Goldstein and Jim Nolan, "Pontiff to Bring Own Blood Supply," *New York Post*, September 10, 1987.

46. Petricciani et al., *AIDS: The Safety of Blood and Blood Products*, p. 27.

47. Associated Press reports, *London Times*, March 20, 1987.

CHAPTER 2
Transfusion History and Practice

1. A. C. Celsus, *De Medecina*, cited in P. Weisz-Carrington, *Principles of Clinical Immunohematology* (Chicago: Year Book Medical Publishers, 1986), p. 1.

2. Ibid.

3. *Encyclopaedia Brittanica*, 15th ed., s.v. "Galen."

4. *Dictionary of Scientific Biography* 6(1972): 152.

5. William Harvey, *De Motu Cordis*, cited in *Dictionary of Scientific Biography* 6(1972): 156.

6. See Louis K. Diamond, "A History of Blood Transfusion," in Maxwell M. Wintrobe, ed., *Blood, Pure and Eloquent* (New York: McGraw-Hill, 1980), p. 662.

7. M. H. Nicholson, *Pepys' Diary and the New Science* (Charlottesville: University of Virginia, 1965), p. 224.

8. Diamond, "Blood Transfusion," p. 663.

9. Ibid.

10. Ibid.

11. Ibid., p. 664.

12. Ibid., p. 668.

13. In 1874 Landois published collected statistics on 478 authenticated transfusions, beginning with Lower and Denis. Landois showed conclusively that animal-to-human transfusions were ill-advised.

14. H. B. Anstall and P. M. Urie, *A Manual of Hemotherapy* (New York: Wiley, 1986), p. 3.

15. T. G. Thomas: "The Intravenous Injection of Milk as a Substitute for the Transfusion of Blood," cited in Diamond, "Blood Transfusion," p. 668.

16. Diamond, "Blood Transfusion," p. 676.

17. Anstall and Urie, *Hemotherapy*, p. 3. Ottenberg also showed that it was safe to transfuse a recipient with blood from a donor whose serum was incompatible with the recipient's red cells, but not the other way around. He was thus the first to make a distinction between "minor-side" cross-match compared with "major-side" cross-match.

18. Diamond, "Blood Transfusion," p. 669.

19. G. W. Crile, *Hemorrhage and Transfusion* (New York and London: Appleton, 1909).

20. *Encyclopaedia Brittanica*, s.v. "blood transfusion."

21. Diamond, "Blood Transfusion," p. 678.

22. Strumia and McGraw had developed a plasma-collection facility as early as 1927. In fact, a wave of enthusiasm for using plasma may have led to some unfortunate catastrophes when it was given in place of whole blood for treatment of shock from blood loss. While its binding proteins make it a better replacement than saline, plasma is no substitute for red cells and can lead to severe anemia.

23. A. W. Drake, S. N. Finkelstein, and H. M. Sapolsky, *The American Blood Supply* (Cambridge, Mass.: MIT Press, 1982), p. 61.

24. Diamond, "Blood Transfusion," p. 683.

25. Andrea Rock, "Inside the Billion-Dollar Business of Blood," *Money*, March 1986, p. 160.

CHAPTER 3

The Blood Supply I:
The Voluntary Sector and Nonprofit Organizations

1. U.S. Congress, *Blood Policy and Technology* (Washington, D.C.: Office of Technology Assessment, 1985), p. 52.

2. Ibid., pp. 52–53. One could argue that the AABB collects 45 percent of the nation's blood supply, since almost all members of the Council of Community Blood Centers belong to the AABB. However, the CCBC is an independent organization that serves its own function and follows separate policies.

3. Ibid.

4. Ibid., p. 51.

5. Andrea Rock, "Inside the Billion-Dollar Business of Blood," *Money*, March 1986. Rock's article also won the Sigma Delta Chi award.

6. Ibid., p. 158.

7. Ibid., p. 158.

8. Ross Eckert, "Blood, Money and Monopoly," in *Securing a Safer Blood Supply: Two Views* (Washington, D.C.: American Enterprise Institute, 1985), p. 33.

9. American Red Cross, Annual Report, 1987: "How We Spend Your Money for Things We Hope You'll Never See," p. 42.

10. A. W. Drake, S. N. Finkelstein, and H. M. Sapolsky, *The American Blood Supply* (Cambridge, Mass.: MIT Press, 1982), pp. 47–48.

11. Ibid., p. 48.

12. Foster Rhea Dulles, *The American Red Cross: A History* (New York: Harper, 1950), pp. 356–57.

13. Eckert, "Blood, Money and Monopoly," p. 37.

14. Dulles, *American Red Cross*, pp. 413–22.

15. Eckert, "Blood, Money and Monopoly," p. 37.

16. Drake, et al., *American Blood Supply*, p. 49.

17. Ibid., p. 50.

18. Ibid., p. 52.

19. U.S. Congress, *Blood Policy and Technology*, p. 52.

20. Drake et al., *American Blood Supply*, pp. 13–21. In Chapter 2, appropriately entitled "Ideologies," the authors provide an excellent discussion of the subject.

21. Ross Eckert, "AIDS and the Blood Bankers," *Regulation*, September/October 1986, p. 16.

22. U.S. Congress, *Blood Policy and Technology*, p. 52.

23. Drake et al., *American Blood Supply*, p. 50.

24. Richard Titmuss, *The Gift Relationship: From Human Blood to Social Policy* (New York: Vintage Books, 1972).

25. Eckert, "Blood, Money and Monopoly," pp. 20–26.

26. Robert M. Solow, "Blood and Thunder," *Yale Law Review* 80 (1971): 1676–1711.

27. Eckert, "Blood, Money and Monopoly," p. 44.

28. Reuben Kessel, "Transfused Blood, Serum Hepatitis and Coase Theorem," *Journal of Law and Economics* 17 (1974): 279–280.

29. Eckert, "AIDS and the Blood Bankers," p. 18.

30. R. Kessel, "Transfused Blood" p. 282.

31. Eckert, "Blood, Money and Monopoly," p. 45.

32. Confirmed in conversation with Andrea Rock, October 22, 1988. A February 1990 article in *The Recorder,* a San Francisco legal newspaper, attacked the American Red Cross for discouraging plaintiffs and their

lawyers with aggressive litigation tactics. The article stated that the Red Cross has a "particularly sinister reputation within the plaintiff bar." One of the attorneys about to try a case against the Red Cross is quoted as saying, "Some of the things they [the Red Cross] did I regard as evil." See "Transfusion-Associated AIDS Cases No 'Pot of Gold,' Attorneys Find," *Blood Bank Week,* February 23, 1990, p. 7.

33. See, for example, "Judge Reverses $1.6 Million Award in AIDS Case," *New York Times,* December 7, 1988; "Blood Bank is Cleared in Colorado AIDS Case," *New York Times,* June 5, 1988; and "Blood Banks Protected under California Law Limiting Damages," *Blood Bank Week,* February 24, 1989.

34. American Blood Commission, *Chronology of the National Blood Policy* (Arlington, Va.: ABC, 1975), p. 2.

35. U.S. Congress, *Blood Policy and Technology,* p. 9.

36. Eckert, "Blood, Money and Monopoly," p. 47.

37. Ibid.

38. Ibid., pp. 49–50.

39. Rock, "Billion-Dollar Business," p. 160.

40. Eckert, "Blood, Money and Monopoly," p. 42.

41. Ibid., p. 43.

42. Unrelated Business Income Tax (UBIT) Hearings before the Subcommittee on Oversight, House Committee on Ways and Means, One Hundredth Congress, Part 1 of 3, Serial 100-26, July 24–26, 1987, p. 2.

CHAPTER 4
The Blood Supply II:
The Plasma Sector and the Role of the Drug Companies

1. U.S. Congress, *Blood Policy and Technology* (Washington, D.C.: Office of Technology Assessment, 1985), p. 63.

2. Ibid., p. 65.

3. Gilbert Gaul, "Plasma Industry to Toughen Rules and Improve Image," *Philadelphial Inquirer,* March 30, 1990.

4. Ross Eckert, "Blood, Money and Monopoly," in *Securing a Safer Blood Supply: Two Views* (Washington, D.C.: American Enterprise Institute, 1985), p. 76.

5. A. W. Drake, S. N. Finkelstein, and H. M. Sapolsky, *The American Blood Supply* (Cambridge, Mass.: MIT, 1982), p. 70.

6. Eckert, "Blood, Money and Monopoly," p. 42.

7. Drake, et al., *American Blood Supply,* p. 62.

8. Eckert, "Blood, Money and Monopoly," p. 6.

9. "The Red Cross: Drawing Blood from Its Rivals," *Business Week*, September 11, 1978, p. 117.

10. Gaul, "Plasma Industry," p. 9.

11. New York Blood Center, Annual Report 1986–87, p. 3.

12. Drake et al., *American Blood Supply,* p. 65.

13. Carol K. Kasper, "Update on AIDS," *The Hemophilia Bulletin,* June 1987, p. 4.

14. New York Blood Center, *Centerpiece,* Winter 1987, p. 5.

15. National Hemophilia Foundation, *Supply Bulletin 11*, March 1989, p. 3.

16. National Hemophilia Foundation, *Supply Bulletin 14,* March 1989.

17. Richard F. Schubert, *Blood Services Bulletin,* quoted by H. Edward Matveld at Unrelated Business Income Tax (UBIT) Hearings before the Subcommittee on Oversight, House Committee on Ways and Means, One Hundredth Congress, June 1987, p. 1077.

18. UBIT Hearings, p. 1078.

19. See Chapter 1, note 22.

20. Andrea Rock, "Inside the Billion-Dollar Business of Blood," *Money,* March 1986, p. 162; and Ross Eckert, "AIDS and the Blood Bankers," *Regulation,* September/October 1986, p. 19.

21. Rock, "Billion-Dollar Business," p. 162.

22. Rock, "Billion-Dollar Business," p. 156.

23. Edgar Engleman, "AIDS and the Blood Supply," *Report of the Presidential Commission on the Human Immunodeficiency Virus Epidemic,* No. 0-214-701 (Washington, D.C.: U.S. Government Printing Office, 1988), p. 4.

24. Rock, "Billion-Dollar Business," p. 156.

25. John Pekkanen, "A Special Report: How Safe Is Our Blood Supply?" *Readers' Digest,* July 1988, p. 39.

CHAPTER 5

The Risks of Transfusion Today

1. Gina Kolata, "New Tests Detect Viral Hepatitis That Is a Threat to Blood Supply," *New York Times,* April 21, 1989, p. 1. The subhead of this article reads, "Transfusions Cause 150,000 Fresh Cases Each Year," referring only to hepatitis non-A, non-B. It is interesting to note that about a year earlier, when the *New York Times* first reported that the test was being developed ("Elusive Hepatitis Virus Reported Isolated," May 11, 1988, p. 1), the figure was even higher: "While estimates vary, Dr. Alter said that about 5 percent, or 200,000 of the 4 million people who undergo transfusions in the United States each year, are exposed to hepatitis non-A, non-B." While some estimates are more than twice as

high ("12% of All Transfused Patients Develop Non-A Non-B Hepatitis," *Obstetrics and Gynecology News,* May 1–14, 1986), it is noteworthy that blood bankers publicly admitted even this (conservative) assessment of the extent of contamination in the nation's blood supply.

2. P. B. Beeson, "Jaundice Occurring One to Four Months after Transfusion of Blood or Plasma," *Journal of the American Medical Association* 121 (1943): 1332.

3. Harold M. Schmeck, Jr., "Researchers Suggest Virus Link to Alzheimer's Disease," *New York Times,* July 23, 1988, p. 11.

4. Lawrence K. Altman, M.D., "Lyme Disease from a Transfusion? It's Unlikely But Experts Are Wary," *New York Times,* July 18, 1989, p. C3.

5. P. L. Mollison, C. P. Engelfriet, and M. Contreras, *Blood Transfusion in Clinical Medicine* (Oxford: Blackwell Scientific Publications, 1987), p. 793.

6. H. B. Anstall and P. M. Urie, *Manual of Hemotherapy* (Wiley, 1986), p. 321.

7. S. Faivelson-Neustein, "Hepatitis B: A Growing Threat," *McCall's,* November 1988, p. 104.

8. Merck Pharmaceuticals, *Bulletin for Hepatitis B Vaccine,* May 1988, p. 2.

9. "12% Develop Hepatitis," p. 3.

10. "CDC Issues Compilation of Anti-Infection Guidelines for Prevention of HBV, HIV in Health Care Workers," *Blood Bank Week,* July 21, 1989, p. 2.

11. Anstall and Urie, *Manual of Hemotherapy,* p. 323.

12. Faivelson-Neustein, p. 104.

13. Anstall and Urie, *Manual of Hemotherapy,* pp. 318–20.

14. Mollison et al., *Blood Transfusion,* p. 774.

15. H. J. Alter, "Post-transfusion Hepatitis: Clinical Features, Risk and Donor Testing," in *Infection, Immunity and Blood Transfusion,* R. Y. Dodd and L. F. Barker (New York: Alan R. Liss, 1985), pp. 47–61.

16. John Pekkanen, "A Special Report: How Safe Is Our Blood Supply?" *Reader's Digest,* July 1988, p. 39.

17. "12% Develop Hepatitis," p. 1.

18. A. W. Drake, S. N. Finkelstein, and H. M. Sapolsky, *The American Blood Supply* (Cambridge, Mass.: MIT Press, 1982), p. 32.

19. Kolata, "New Tests," p. 1.

20. "Medical Research: Protecting Profits or Patients? ABC News Nightline," Show No. 2065, April 21, 1989, Transcript by Journal Graphics, Inc., April 27, 1989, p. 5.

21. Since the earliest, optimistic forecasts that the new test would eliminate most non-A, non-B hepatitis from the blood supply, there has already been a significant revision downward. New evidence suggests that only

about one-half of the cases of non-A, non-B hepatitis may be detected by the hepatitis C test. There are many other viruses—soon there will surely be one called non-A, non-B, non-C hepatitis—that will not be picked up. See "Study Shows HCV Responsible for Half of NANB Hepatitis Cases," *Blood Bank Week*, January 12, 1990, p. 1.

22. Kolata, "New Tests," p. 1. As mentioned earlier (see Chapter 1, note 3, and Chapter 5, note 1), these figures are low estimates.

23. "Medical Research: Protecting Profits or Patients?" Transcript, p. 2 (Bonnie Strauss).

24. T. B. Wallington, "Cytomegalovirus and Transfusion," in John D. Cash, ed., *Progress in Transfusion Medicine*, vol. 2 (Edinburgh & New York: Churchill Livingstone, 1987), p. 27.

25. Mollison et al., *Blood Transfusion*, p. 794.

26. Ibid., p. 795.

27. Wallington, "Cytomegalovirus and Transfusion," p. 35.

28. "Hemorrhage Can Suppress Immune System," *American Medical News*, January 23–30, 1987, p. 51.

29. Wallington, "Cytomegalovirus and Transfusion," p. 28.

30. Mollison et al., *Blood Transfusion*, p. 794.

31. Edgar Engleman, "AIDS and the Blood Supply," *Report to the Presidential Commission on the Human Immunodeficiency Virus Epidemic*, No. 0-214-701 (Washington, D.C.: U.S. Government Printing Office, 1988), pp. 6–7.

32. Ross Eckert, "AIDS and the Blood Bankers," *Regulation*, September/October 1986, p. 18.

33. Wallington, "Cytomegalovirus and Transfusion," p. 31.

34. J. P. Ibister and D. H. Pittiglio *Clinical Hematology* (Baltimore: Williams & Wilkins, 1988), p. 211.

35. Harold M. Schmeck, Jr., "Red Cross Plans to Test for Rare Virus Tied to Cancer," *New York Times*, April 29, 1988, p. 1.

36. M. Robert-Guroff, S. H. Weiss, J. A. Giron, A. M. Jennings, H. M. Ginsburg, I. B. Margolis, W. A. Blattner, and R. C. Gallo, "Prevalence of Antibodies to HTLV-I, -II, and -III in Intravenous Drug Abusers from an AIDS Endemic Region," *Journal of the American Medical Association* 255 (1986): 3133–37.

37. "HTLV-II Prevalent among Drug Addicts in Major U.S. Cities," *Blood Bank Week*, February 24, 1989, p. 5.

38. Mollison et al., *Blood Transfusion*, p. 799. Ross Eckert also argues for syphilis testing in his "Statement on Blood Safety," *Report of Presidential Commission*.

39. Eckert, "Statement on Blood Safety," pp. 4–5.

40. Mollison et al., *Blood Transfusion*, p. 802.

41. Bruce Lambert, "4 Cases Found of Rare Strain of AIDS Virus," *New York Times,* June 27, 1989, p. 81.

42. Ibid.

43. Lawrence K. Altman, M.D., "Scientists Fear That a Parasite Will Spread in Transfusions," *New York Times,* May 23, 1989, p. C3.

44. Ibid.

45. Mollison et al., *Blood Transfusion,* p. 800.

46. Larry Thompson, "Doctors Take Another Look at Transfusions," *Washington Post Health,* July 5, 1988, p. 6.

47. J. C. Barton, "Nonhemolytic, Noninfectious Transfusion Reactions," *Seminars in Hematology* 18 (1981): 95.

48. Thompson, "Doctors Take Another Look," p. 6.

CHAPTER 6
AIDS: A Special Case

1. CDC, "Kaposi's Sarcoma and *Pneumocystis* Pneumonia among Homosexual Men—New York and California," *Morbidity and Mortality Weekly* 30 (1981): 305–8.

2. CDC and Surgeon General, "Understanding AIDS," No. 532-152 (Washington, D.C.: U.S. Government Printing Office, 1988) p. 3.

3. L. Resnick et al., "Stability and Inactivation of HTLV-III/LAV under Clinical and Laboratory Environments," *Journal of the American Medical Association* 255 (1986): 1887–91.

4. M. Piazza et al., "Passionate Kissing and Microlesions of the Oral Mucosa: Possible Role in AIDS Transmission" (Letter), *Journal of the American Medical Association* 261, no. 2 (1989).

5. Ibid.

6. "Test Developed to Detect HIV in Saliva," *Blood Bank Week,* April 28, 1989, p. 3.

7. "Number of HIV-Infected Workers Underestimated," *Blood Bank Week,* January 19, 1990, p. 2.

8. Ibid. Some of the reasons for underreporting include fear on the part of doctors and nurses that they will lose their jobs if they contract HIV, and fear on the part of hospitals that patients will go elsewhere if they learn a staff member is infected. Critics charge that the CDC also contributes to the low totals by using overly stringent criteria for determining which infections were caused by workplace exposures as contrasted with social exposures. The CDC has also reportedly moved too slowly in investigation.

9. *Blood Bank Week,* February 19, 1988, p. 3, addresses the U.S. Public Health Service figures. See also *Report of the Presidential Commission on the*

Human Immunodeficiency Virus Epidemic, No. 0-214-701 (Washington, D.C.: U.S. Government Printing Office, 1988) p. XVII.

10. Philip M. Boffey, "Research Group Says AIDS Cases May Be Twice the U. S. Estimate," *New York Times,* August 20, 1988, p. 1.

11. W. H. Masters, V. E. Johnson, and R. C. Kolodney, *Crisis: Heterosexual Behavior in the Age of AIDS* (New York: Grove Press, 1988), pp. 3–4.

12. Ibid., p. 4.

13. Boffey, "Research Group and AIDS Estimate," p. 1.

14. Ibid.

15. "Complacency Seen in Battle on AIDS," *New York Times,* November 3, 1989, p. 18.

16. David T. Imagawa et al., "Human Immunodeficiency Virus Type 1 Infection in Homosexual Men Who Remain Seronegative for Prolonged Periods," *New England Journal of Medicine* 320 (1989): 1458–62.

17. S. Z. Salahuddin et al., HTLV III in Symptom Free Seronegative Persons," *Lancet* ii (December 1984): 1418.

18. *Report of Presidential Commission,* p. XVIII. A later estimate put the average period between infection with AIDS and the onset of symptoms at 10 years. Lawrence K. Altman, "Who's Stricken and How: AIDS Pattern Is Shifting," *New York Times,* February 5, 1989, p. 1. The CDC estimates that about 120,000, or fewer than 10%, of the 1.4 million people believed to be infected with AIDS have been tested and are aware of their condition.

19. In a 1987 University of California study that looked back at transfusion recipients who had received blood between 1978 and 1985, about 1 in 50 was positive for AIDS, while another 2% were unconfirmed antibody positive. At that time, 2.5% had died of transfusion-related AIDS. Perhaps most remarkable of all, 12% did not even realize they had received a transfusion. See Elizabeth Donegan et al., Letter to the Editor, "Mass Notification of Transfusion Recipients at Risk for HIV Infection," *Journal of the American Medical Association* 260 (August 1988): 922–23.

20. *Report of the Presidential Commission on HIV,* p. 78.

21. Gina Kolata, "Study Claims AIDS Virus May Be Latent for a Year," *New York Times,* October 3, 1987, p. 1. "Because people at high risk of AIDS are told not to donate blood and because of the extremely sensitive screening tests, fewer than *one in 250,000* transfusions are now contaminated, according to federal estimates" (italics added).

22. Ibid. "The finding also raises new questions about the potential effectiveness of proposed mass screening programs for carriers of the virus that causes acquired immune deficiency syndrome. Blood bank officials, however, stressed the supply of blood products for medical use remained *extremely safe*" (italics added). See also CDC, "Human Immuno-

deficiency Virus Infection in Transfusion Recipients and Their Family Members," *Morbidity and Mortality Weekly Report* 36, no. 10 (1987): 1861, where a characteristic claim reads: "The risk of HIV transmission by transfusion was low, even before screening, and has been *virtually eliminated* by the routine screening of donated blood and plasma" (italics added). These claims have been picked up and repeated by all blood banking organizations and by the media.

23. Paul D. Cummings et al., "Exposure of Patients to Human Immunodeficiency Virus Through the Transfusion of Blood Components That Test Antibody-Negative," *New England Journal of Medicine* (1989): 941–46.
24. Ibid., p. 941.
25. Alan Salzberg et al., Letter to the Editor, *New England Journal of Medicine* 319 (August 1988): 515. Although Salzberg has since modified his estimates about San Francisco, he still believes that cities like New York carry a much higher risk of HIV in the blood supply than do low-risk areas (verbal communication with Alan Salzberg, October 22, 1989).
26. Robert Steinbrook, "Transfusion AIDS Risk Scaled Back," *Los Angeles Times*, October 5, 1989, p. 38.
27. Cummings et al., "Exposure to HIV," p. 941.
28. S. Wolinsky et al., "Polymerase Chain Reaction (PCR) Detection of HIV Provirus Before HIV Seroconversion," paper presented at the fourth international conference on AIDS, Stockholm, June 12–16, 1988 (abstract).
29. Imagawa et al., "HIV-1 in Homosexual Men."
30. Cummings et al., "Exposure to HIV," p. 942.
31. Steinbrook, "Scaled Back"; see also John W. Ward et al., "The Natural History of Transfusion-Associated Infection with Human Immunodeficiency Virus," *New England Journal of Medicine* 321 (October 1989): 947–52.
32. *Report of Presidential Commission*, p. 78.
33. " 'Healthy HIV Seropositive' Said to Be a Misnomer," *Internal Medicine News,* January 15–31, 1989.
33A. "Studies Measure Levels of HIV in Infected Blood," *Blood Bank Week,* December 15, 1989. The levels of infectious HIV in blood were much higher than previously estimated.
34. Chris Corcoran, "Anti-AIDS Group Assails Ad for Blood Donors in Gay Newspaper," *New York Tribune,* May 10, 1988.
35. Ibid.
36. Allen White, "Leaders Urge Donors: 'Write Protest Letters to Irwin Blood Bank,' "*Bay Area Reporter,* August 1, 1988. Karen Everett, "Community Blood Drives Reinstated in Castro," *San Francisco Sentinel,* August 19, 1988.

37. See Chapter 1, note 38.

38. D. B. Barnes, "New Questions about AIDS Test Accuracy," *Science* 238 (1987): 884–85.

39. Tinker Ready, "Contamination Prompts Review at Blood Centers," *HealthWeek,* April 11, 1988.

40. Robert Manor and Fred W. Lindecke, "Blood Given to Six Might Be AIDS-Tainted," *St. Louis Post-Dispatch,* July 28, 1988.

41. See *Blood Bank Week,* vol. 5: no. 13, p. 1, no. 16, p. 1; and no. 27, p. 1.

42. J. N. Weber et al., "Human Immunodeficiency Virus in Two Cohorts of Homosexual Men: Neutralizing Sera and Association of Anti-gag Antibody with Prognosis," *Lancet* 1 (January 1987): 119–22.

43. G. Ujhelyi et al., "Studies of the Sensitivity and Reproducibility of Commercial Kits to Detect Antibodies to Human Immunodeficiency Virus," *Transfusion* 27 (1987): 210–12.

44. J. R. Carlson et al., "AIDS Serology Testing in low- and high-risk groups," *Journal of the American Medical Association* 253 (1985): 3405–8.

45. A. J. Saah et al., "Detection of Early Antibodies in Human Immunodeficiency Virus Infection by Enzyme-Linked immunosorbent assay, Western blot and Radoiimunoprecipitation," *Journal of Clinical Microbiology* 25 (1987): 1605–10.

46. Susan L. Stramer et al., "Markers of HIV Infection Prior to IgG Antibody Seropositivity," *Journal of the American Medical Association* 262 (July 1989): 64–69. It is significant that the plasma donors in this study did not come from high-prevalence coastal areas. The infected donors also filled out a questionnaire on risk behavior, and those in high-risk categories were excluded. In this study, neither prescreening nor self-deferral was an effective deterrent.

47. Gina Kolata, "AIDS Virus Found to Hide in Cells, Eluding Detection by Normal Tests," *New York Times,* June 5, 1988.

48. Imagawa et al., "HIV-1 in Homosexual Men."

49. Even Gina Kolata, one of the better science reporters for the *New York Times,* created a misleading impression in a front-page article published June 1, 1989. Kolata talked about "one quarter of a group of homosexual men" as if they were the ones who slipped through the test. In fact, about one-quarter, or 31 out of 133, were infected with AIDS. But of these 31, all but 4, or 87%, slipped through the standard AIDS test and did not show up positive for three years or more! Later in the article, Kolata quotes Dr. Jaffe and Dr. Sininsky as saying that "they did not expect that a quarter of all people who were exposed to the virus and tested negative on the antibody test actually were infected." Once again, this one-quarter figure is misleading. The shocking finding was that of those who were infected with AIDS, the vast majority, or 27 out of 31,

were not being detected by the test. See Gina Kolata, "AIDS Test May Fail to Detect Virus for Years, Study Finds," *New York Times,* June 1, 1989, and compare with the actual *New England Journal of Medicine* study by Imagawa et al., "HIV-1 in Homosexual Men."

50. Imagawa et al., "HIV-1 in Homosexual Men," p. 1461.

51. Ibid., pp. 1458–59.

52. Alan Salzberg et al., Letter to Editor, p. 515.

53. See, for example, Corcoran, "Anti-AIDS Group Assails Ad."

54. Salzberg et al., Letter to Editor.

55. James R. Allen, "Epidemiologic Considerations in the Transmission of LAV/HTLV-III by Blood and Blood Products," in *AIDS: The Safety of Blood and Blood Products,* ed. J. C. Petricciani et al. (New York: Wiley, 1987), p. 38.

56. John Pekkanen, "How Safe Is Our Blood Supply?" *Reader's Digest,* July 1988.

57. Lloyd F. Novick et al., "HIV Seroprevalence in Newborns in New York State, *Journal of the American Medical Association* 261 (March 1989): 1745.

58. Noah D. Cohen et al., "Transmission of Retroviruses by Transfusion of Screened Blood in Patients Undergoing Cardiac Surgery," *New England Journal of Medicine* 320 (May 1989): 1172–76.

59. Verbal communication from Alan Salzberg, October 22, 1989. Salzberg believes that new drugs like AZT—which slow the progression of AIDS without eliminating it—may create a misleading impression that there are fewer new cases. Like many AIDS experts, he believes that more data are needed to ascertain the true extent of the epidemic.

60. Masters et al., *Crisis,* p. 78.

61. "FDA and CDC: 6-Month Quarantine for AIDS," *American Association of Tissue Banks Newsletter,.* vol. 11, February 1988, p. 1.

62. Ward et al., "The Natural History of Transfusion-Associated HIV."

63. FDA memorandum, "Subject: Recommendations for Changeover from Use of Fresh Immunizing Red Blood Cells to Use of Frozen Immunizing Red Blood Cells Stored a Minimum of Six Months Prior to Use," *Plamaspheresis,* November 1988, p. 264.

64. "Heterosexual Partners of Persons with HIV Infection at Recognized Risk," *AABB Blood Bank Week,* February 19, 1988. The risk for heterosexual partners is placed between 10% and 60%.

65. "AIDS-Infected Marine Sues U.S. over Transfusion of Tainted Blood," *New York Times,* June 22, 1988.

66. "Transfusion-Associated AIDS Is Subject of Network TV," *Blood Bank Week,* February 23, 1990.

67. "Revision of Definition of AIDS Yields Jump in Reported Cases," April

28, 1989, p. 2. Among women, 11% of those infected with HIV have histories of blood transfusion.

68. Kolata, "Study Claims AIDS Virus May Be Latent," p. 1.

69. Kolata, "AIDS Test May Fail to Detect Virus," p. 1.

CHAPTER 7

Undertransfusion

1. See "Mystery of Manes' Missing 7 Hours," *New York Post,* January 11, 1986, p. 3.

2. As reported in "Manes in Coronary Unit: Borough President Moved after Suffering Chest Pains," *Daily News,* January 12, 1986, p. 5.

3. P. L. Mollison et al., *Blood Transfusion in Clinical Medicine* (Boston: Blackwell Scientific Publications, 1987), p. 68.

4. Ibid., p. 46.

5. Ibid.

6. Such studies include, for example, "Do Running and Blood Donating Mix?" *The Physician and Sportsmedicine* 16, no. 7 (1988): 30; also Robert F. Weiss, "The Dope on Blood Doping," *Greenwich [Connecticut] News,* December 7, 1989, p. 2.

7. While a figure of five one-unit donations in five weeks is often cited, AABB guidelines theoretically permit even more blood to be drawn for autologous use. "Donations are often scheduled weekly or even at four-day intervals, with the last phlebotomy performed 72 hours or more before the operation." Council on Scientific Affairs, "Autologous Blood Transfusions," *Journal of the American Medical Association* 256 (November 1986): 2378.

8. According to a recent study comparing autologous blood donors undergoing elective orthopedic surgery and a matched group who were not autologous blood donors, "physicians accepted lower hematocrit levels for autologous blood-donor patients at all points during the surgical hospitalization, which suggests that physicians lower their 'transfusion trigger' hematocrit levels for patients who deposit autologous blood." See Alan L. Hull et al., "Effects of a CME Program on Physicians' Transfusion Practices," *Academic Medicine* 64 (1989): 681–85.

9. "Patients did not store sufficient amounts of autologous blood to minimize their exposure to homologous blood, as demonstrated by the fact that 30 units of homologous blood were transfused in addition to the 107 autologous units." Ibid., p. 683.

10. See the standard guidelines in P. V. Holland and P. J. Schmidt, eds., *Standards for Blood Banks and Transfusion Services,* 12th ed. (Arlington, Va.: American Association of Blood Banks, 1987).

11. Thomas S. Kickler and Jerry L. Spivak, "Effect of Repeated Whole Blood Donations on Serum Immunoreactive Erythropoietin Levels in Autologous Donors," *Journal of the American Medical Association* 260 (July 1988): 65–67. The April 1989 edition of *Archives of Surgery* reported that many patients who wished to receive autologous blood were unable to do so because they could not replenish their red cell supplies between phlebotomies. Reported in *Blood Bank Week,* April 29, 1989, p. 5.

12. See, for example, William C. Schraft, "Saving Our Blood Supply," *The New York Doctor,* October 31, 1988, p. 28.

13. Ibid. See also Holland and Schmidt, eds., *Standards for Blood Banks,* p. 4.

14. Holland and Schmidt, eds., *Standards for Blood Banks,* p. 39.

15. "Do Running and Blood Donating Mix?" pp. 30, 32. "After four and eight weeks, the blood donors approached or equalled their original three-mile run times. This seems to indicate that their running was back to normal within four weeks" (p. 30).

16. National Institutes of Health Consensus, "Blood Transfusion: The State of the Art," *Emergency Medicine,* November 30, 1988. While explaining the "10/30" rule, the article admits that there is very little solid, scientific data on which to base it: "However, the literature is remarkable for the absence of carefully controlled randomized trials that would permit definitive conclusions regarding perioperative transfusion practices" (p. 182).

17. Jeffrey L. Carlson et al. "Severity of Anaemia and Operative Mortality and Morbidity," *Lancet* i (April 1988): 727–29.

18. "Quality of Life in End-Stage Renal Disease Found Greatly Improved with Erythropoietin," *Internal Medicine News* 22 no. 23 (December 1989): 3.

19. Ibid.

20. Weiss, "The Dope on Blood Doping."

21. Michael O'Connor, "U.S. Skier Admits to Bloodpacking," *Boston Herald,* December 30, 1987, p. 30.

22. New York Blood Center, Public Information Department, "Some Facts about Blood Transfusions," New York, 1988. The 12% figure includes all injuries, including those sustained at home. Although there are no precise figures, the number of injuries resulting from car accidents is probably less than half of this total, accounting for under 5% of all blood transfusions.

23. Carlson et al., "Severity of Anaemia."

24. "Hemorrhage can Suppress Immune System," *American Medical News,* January 23/30, 1987, p. 51. Mice who were exposed to infection after being bled had almost twice the mortality rate of controls not subjected to hemorrhage. Since blood loss alone was enough to suppress the immune system, the study concluded that any additional trauma would

be expected to have an additive effect. One can easily understand why patients facing the trauma of surgery should have a full supply of blood.

CHAPTER 8
The Blood Bank of the Future

1. Susan Jenks, "Case Builds Against Transfusions," *Medical World News*, December 11, 1989, p. 28. Receiving blood from an outside source has long been known to temporarily weaken one's immune system. Two doctors from the University of Rochester, Dr. Johanna Heal and Dr. Neil Blumberg, recently became the first in the country to look at the effects of autologous blood transfusions on immunosuppression and postoperative infection. Comparing rates of infection among hip replacement patients following surgery, the researchers found that 23% of those who received homologous blood contracted an infection, while those patients who received their own blood or were not transfused had no infection postoperatively at all.

2. See Chapter 1, note 42.

3. See Chapter 1, note 26.

4. Although intraoperative salvage can save as much as 50% of the blood required for transfusion in certain specialized cases—*Journal of the American Medical Association* 256 (November 1986): 2379—it does not have a significant impact on overall need for blood. See, for example, William C. Schraft, "Saving Our Blood Supply," *The New York Doctor*, October 31, 1988. "We have had the cell saver for about two years and estimate that this saves up to 3 percent of our transfused blood, but no more" (p. 28).

5. Jill A. Davis, "Doctor Studies Ways to Make Blood Supplies Safer," *Marblehead [Mass.] Reporter*, January 12, 1989. The article deals with the work of Dr. C. Robert Valeri, one of the pioneers of long-term preservation of blood, who is the scientific director of the Naval Blood Research Laboratory. "He [Dr. Valeri] said the Navy is able to freeze red blood cells up to 21 years, and likely even longer, at −80 degrees. At this point, the Food and Drug Administration has only approved the freezing of red blood cells up to 10 years" (p. 1).

6. L. L. Haynes et al., "Clinical Use of Glycerolized Frozen Blood," *Journal of the American Medical Association* 173 (1960): 1657. See also C. R. Valeri et al., "Therapeutic effectiveness of homologous erythrocyte transfusions following frozen storage at −80 for up to 7 years," *Transfusion* 10 (1970): 102. Haynes found that red cells stored from 3 to 4 years had a posttransfusion survival of 95%. After 7 years, Valeri showed survival of 90% in red cells. The only drawback of frozen blood is that it must be used within 24 hours of being thawed.

7. Private communication from Dr. Denis Goldfinger and Dr. Frederick

Axlerod, blood bank directors of Cedars of Sinai Hospital in Los Angeles, April 15, 1989.

8. "We believe that two specific messages are given to the physician by the autologous donor: (1) the patient believes that the likelihood of needing blood during surgery is high (that is, blood has a benefit); and (2) the patient is aware of the risks of using homologous blood and proposes a process to retain the benefits of blood transfusion while reducing the risks. These messages probably cause the physician to behave differently with the autologous-blood-donor patient than with other patients." Alan L. Hull et al., "Effects of a CME Program on Physicians' Transfusion Practices," *Academic Medicine* 64 (1989): 682.

9. Even the American Red Cross has subsequently acknowledged the importance of keeping the number of donors to a minimum. "Physicians should also be aware that the risk of HIV is likely to be lower if products from fewer donors are involved; the transfusion of one unit of pheresed platelets is preferable to that of six or eight units from random donors." Paul D. Cummings et al., "Exposure of Patients to Human Immunodeficiency Virus Through the Transfusion of Blood Components that Test Antibody-Negative," *New England Journal of Medicine* 321 (October 1989): 944.

10. John Henahan, "Perfluorocarbon 'Blood' Flops in U.S. Trials," *Medical Tribune,* March 18, 1987, p. 1.

11. Ibid.

12. J. I. Mathews et al., "Photodynamic Therapy of Viral Contaminants with Potential for Blood Banking Applications," *Transfusion* 28, no. 1 (1988): 81–83.

13. See Bruce Lambert, "FDA Gives Quick Approval to Two Drugs to Treat AIDS," *New York Times,* June 27, 1989, p. 1.

14. Sales of erythropoietin have soared as athletes have discovered its ability to significantly improve performance. See Laura Jereshin, "It Gives Athletes a Boost—Maybe Too Much," *Business Week,* December 11, 1989, p. 123.

15. Andrea Rock, "Inside the Billion-Dollar Business of Blood," *Money,* March 1986, p. 169.

16. R. R. Corden et al., "Experience with 11,916 Designated Donors," *Transfusion* 26 (1986): 484–86.

17. Debra Lynn Vial, "Blood Bank Tourniquet," *Fairfax Journal,* December 21, 1988.

Glossary

AABB. American Association of Blood Banks. One of the two main blood banking organizations, a trade group that functions as the major accrediting agency in the United States for blood bank standards.

agglutination. A reaction in which particles such as red blood cells collect into clumps. Agglutination can be caused by multiple factors, among them antibodies.

AIDS. An acronym for acquired immune deficiency syndrome. A disease pattern caused by a special retrovirus that destroys the immune system of the body.

ALT. An acronym for alanine aminotransferase, a liver enzyme normally present in the blood. When the liver is damaged, as in hepatitis, increased amounts of this enzyme are found in the blood.

American Red Cross. The largest blood-collecting agency in the United States, a not-for-profit organization that also engages in war and disaster relief.

anaphylaxis. A severe immunologic reaction involving the complete collapse of the circulation.

anastomosis. The process of surgically connecting two blood vessels to one another.

anemia. A condition in which the blood is deficient in red blood cells, in hemoglobin, or in total volume. In a man a hematocrit under 40 is considered anemic; in a woman, 36 and under.

angiography. An X-ray study of blood vessels using a dye that is injected into the vessels and that reveals the degree of blockage.

antibodies. Special proteins found in the blood which help white cells neutralize foreign invaders such as viruses and bacteria. Antibodies are a key part of the immune system.

anticoagulant. A chemical substance that prevents the clotting of blood.

antigens. Any foreign proteins or substances which stimulate the production of antibodies when introduced into the body. For example, different parts of invading bacteria or a virus are antigens to which the body produces antibodies as a countermeasure.

arteriosclerosis. A condition in which the arteries of the body become stiff-ened and lined with abnormal cholesterol and calcium deposits.

artery. One of the branching vessels that carry blood from the heart through the body.

artificial blood (also called *synthetic blood*). Compounds or chemicals artifi-cially made whose primary function is to carry oxygen.

atrium. One of the two main collecting chambers of the heart.

autologous transfusion (also called *self-storage* or *self-donation*). Transfusion with one's own blood that has previously been donated and stored.

bacteria. Small organisms that can live and reproduce either inside or out-side the body, wherever appropriate conditions exist.

blood banking. The practice of storing blood with a preservative for future use.

blood brokers. Individuals or groups who buy and sell blood products. Among the largest blood brokers in the United States is the American Red Cross.

blood cleansing. Removing infectious organisms from blood by various means. To date, no method has been found to cleanse blood totally of impurities and retain its usability.

blood clotting. The ability of the blood to coagulate and stop flowing out.

blood components. The basic elements into which blood is broken down, in-cluding red cells, white cells, plasma, and platelets. Plasma is further subdivided into multiple blood products called blood derivatives.

blood group. One of the classes into which human beings can be separated on the basis of the presence or absence in their blood of specific antigens. There are four major blood groups—A, B, AB, and O—and about 600 blood subtypes. In common parlance *blood group* is often used interchange-ably with *blood type.*

blood loss. The amount of blood lost, in practice often difficult to measure in exact quantities. The hematocrit (q.v.) is frequently used as a measure of how much blood an individual is missing.

blood matching. Tests performed on blood to determine the various types and subtypes contained within a person's blood.

blood product. A substance made from blood which may be used either for treatment or for diagnostic purposes.

blood replacement. The replenishing of a patient's blood loss.

blood supply. The amount of blood that is stored in various blood banks across the country and is available for transfusion.

blood type. See *blood group.*

blood vessels. The veins, arteries, and capillaries.

blood volume. A measurement of the total amount of blood that an individual has in his or her body.

capillary. One of the minute blood vessels that connect the smallest arteries with the smallest veins. It is at the site of the capillaries that the key exchange of oxygen and carbon dioxide takes place.

CCBC. Council of Community Blood Centers. The third and smallest of the major blood banking organizations in the United States.

CDC. (U.S.) Centers for Disease Control. The major federal organization which collects and coordinates information and research on disease in the United States.

cell saver. A machine that collects and filters blood for reinfusion during surgery.

Chagas' disease. A widespread disease in South America transmitted by a parasite, it causes an incurable form of heart disease. It has recently been reported to be transmitted by blood transfusions given in the United States.

chemotherapy. The use of chemical agents to treat various forms of cancer. The aim is to find a chemical substance that destroys malignant tissue and leaves healthy tissue undamaged.

cirrhosis. A potentially fatal condition of the liver in which liver cells are destroyed and replaced by nonfunctioning scar tissue.

commercial blood. See *paid blood.*

cross-coverage. With respect to blood, the extra protection one gets when compatible blood is pooled and stored by a group of people for their common use.

cryobiology. The science that deals with preservation of tissues by freezing at ultra-low temperatures.

cryopreservation. Preservation of biological materials, such as blood or plasma, at very low temperatures.

culture. Living matter grown in a prepared medium. Foreign organisms are often identified by placing a sample of blood or other fluid in growth media that enable the organisms to multiply outside the body.

cytomegalovirus (CMV). A contagious viral disease which in some humans causes multiple symptoms. While about half of the population has been exposed to this virus without developing serious disease, it can cause severe illness, including hepatitis, when contracted through a blood transfusion.

defibrinated blood. Blood from which some of the key clotting elements have been removed.

detectability. The degree to which something can be found. Certain diseases may be present in the body but undetectable by standard tests.

directed donation (also called *designated donation*). Blood donated and earmarked for a specific person, as opposed to blood donated for the general supply.

ELISA. Enzyme-linked immunosorbent assay. Among the tests using this technique are the screening tests used to detect AIDS antibodies.

endocrinology. The science of glandular function.

Epstein-Barr virus (EBV). A virus that may cause hepatitis and other widespread infections, such as mononucleosis, that can linger for years. Despite its infectivity, EBV is not screened for in blood.

erythropoietin. A hormone that stimulates the bone marrow to reproduce red blood cells. It is now produced by genetic engineering for treatment of anemic patients.

Euroblood. Whole blood that is collected in Europe and shipped to the United States.

exchange transfusion. Removal of a patient's blood and replacement with other blood.

Factor VIII. Plasma derivative that is essential in helping blood clot. The factor is missing in most hemophiliacs, who are treated with Factor VIII, manufactured from human blood.

FDA. Food and Drug Administration. The main federal agency which approves pharmaceutical drugs and helps sets standards for blood banks.

fibrinogen. A derivative of fractionated plasma that contains an important clotting factor.

fractionation. The separation of plasma into useful blood derivatives.

fresh-frozen plasma. Plasma removed and frozen without preservatives within hours after collection.

frozen blood. Blood that can be stored indefinitely at super-low temperatures with the help of a preservative.

gamma globulin. A derivative of blood plasma that contains valuable antibodies against viruses and bacteria.

glycerol. A special fat used as a preservative or antifreeze in long-term freezing and preservation of blood.

heart attack. The destruction of a segment of the heart due to inadequate blood flow.

hemapheresis. The process whereby only a desired blood component is taken from the donor's blood and the remaining fluid and blood cells are immediately transfused back.

hematocrit. The percentage of blood that consists of red blood cells, measured by spinning down a blood sample in a centrifuge. (The remaining portion of the blood is called the *plasma.*) The hematocrit is one of the most basic measurements performed by physicians to determine whether adequate blood is present in an individual.

hematologist. A physician who specializes in diseases involving the blood.

hemodilution. A process of collecting the patient's blood prior to an operation and retransfusing it during surgery to minimize exposure.

hemolysis. The destruction or rupture of the blood cells and the release of the contents of the red cells into the bloodstream.

hemophilia. A hereditary disease caused by the absence of clotting factors in the blood. There are two major types, hemophilia A and B, and they both predominantly affect men.

hemorrhage. Extensive bleeding.

hemorrhagic shock. A condition in which an individual loses so much blood that vital areas of the body are deprived of oxygen. Shock accompanies 70 to 80 percent of battle wounds.

hepatitis. An inflammation of the liver from multiple causes such as viruses and bacteria, as well as chemicals like alcohol. About one in ten people receiving blood transfusions develops hepatitis.

hepatitis B core antibody test. A test that detects antibodies at the core of the hepatitis B virus and thus indicates past exposure to hepatitis B.

hepatitis C. A tentative new name for one of the viruses causing non-A, non-B hepatitis.

HIV. Human immunodeficiency virus, the infectious agent implicated as the cause of AIDS.

homologous blood. Blood donated from another person, as opposed to autologous blood which is donated to oneself. See also *autologous transfusion.*

immune. Having or producing antibodies to a corresponding antigen.

immune system. The combination of all cells and compounds produced by the body to fight disease.

immunosuppressed. A condition in which the immune system has been damaged.

inactivation (also called *deactivation*). A method of killing infectious organisms while retaining important properties of a blood component.

incidence. The frequency or rate of occurrence of any event over a period of time in relation to the population in which it occurs. Compare *prevalence.*

incompatibility. A situation in which the mixing of blood from two different individuals leads to destruction of blood components.

infarction. The destruction of an organ or part of an organ because of insufficient blood flow.

infectious agent. A foreign substance, such as a bacterium or a virus, capable of reproducing itself within the body.

intraoperative salvage. A process in which a patient's blood lost during surgery is collected, washed, and reinfused as soon as possible through a machine sometimes known as a *cell saver.*

latent infection. Hidden infection kept in check by a healthy body.

leukemia. A form of blood cell cancer.

leukocyte. See *white blood cells.*

look-back program. A retrospective study that attempts to identify recipients of blood from a donor later found to be HIV-antibody positive.

Lyme disease. A disease caused by a spirochete which may cause arthritis and other severe impairments. It is usually spread by a bite from a tick but can also be transmitted through blood transfusions.

lymphadenopathy. An enlargement of the lymph nodes, frequently associated with disease. It can be an early sign of AIDS.

lymphoma. A form of cancer.

macrophage. One of the white blood cells involved in fighting bacteria. It has been shown to harbor the AIDS virus.

malaria. One of the most widespread diseases in the world, caused by a parasite. It is rarely seen in the United States but can be spread by blood.

monodonor. A single donor who provides several blood components, especially platelets, to a transfusion recipient, thus minimizing the risk of infection.

NIH. National Institutes of Health.

not-for-profit. The legal definition of certain companies that do not pay taxes because they are intended to serve the public good.

obstetrics. The branch of medicine that relates to the care of pregnant women and childbirth.

opportunistic infection. An infection caused by an organism that rarely causes disease in persons with normal immune systems but attacks those with compromised immunity, such as AIDS patients.

paid blood (also called *commercial blood*). Blood obtained from donors who are paid a fee for donating it. If the donors are adequately screened, this blood is not inferior and may actually be superior to voluntary or unpaid blood.

perfusion. A flow of fluid or blood to nourish a section of the body.

phlebotomy. The active removal of blood from the body.

plasma. The watery part of the blood in which are suspended all the proteins and cells of the bloodstream.

plasma donors. Individuals who donate plasma. Most plasma donors are paid a fee for their blood.

plasmapheresis. A method of removing blood from an individual and separating it into plasma and red cells, and subsequently returning the red cells to the donor.

plasma pool. Plasma that is pooled or mixed together for greater efficiency in processing. A single "pool" is made up of thousands of different donations and, unless the entire pool is sterilized, a single infected donation may contaminate the entire pool.

platelets. Small cells within the bloodstream that are essential for clot formation.

postoperative salvage. A process to recapture profuse blood lost after surgery, using the same technique as intraoperative salvage.

prevalence. The extent of spread, or the number of cases, of a disease present in a specified population at a given time.

quarantine. To separate from contact with others. In the case of a blood sample, it can also mean to hold a specimen in isolation for a specified time until it can be released for safety purposes.

reagent. With reference to blood banking, a substance usually derived from blood itself which is used for testing other blood. For example, reagents used to type blood are made from blood donated by others.

red blood cells. The major cells of the bloodstream. Their primary function is to carry oxygen and remove carbon dioxide.

retrovirus. One of a group of viruses that reproduce by the use of RNA, as opposed to most viruses, which reproduce by copying from DNA. Retroviruses reproduce by taking over the reproductive mechanism within the cell of the host.

Rh factor. Any of one or more inherited substances present in red blood cells and capable of inducing an intense antigenic reaction. When present, an individual is designated *Rh positive,* and when absent, *Rh negative.*

saline solution. A sterile salt solution frequently used as a blood substitute in the initial stages of transfusion.

screening test. A preliminary test to detect a disease or condition. Sometimes requires a follow-up or more specific confirmatory test.

seroconversion. The initial appearance of antibodies in response to a specific antigen that is usually part of the coating of the invading virus or bacteria. Some AIDS patients may harbor the disease for months or even years before they seroconvert (produce antibodies).

seropositive. A condition in which specific antibodies are found in the blood.

serum. The watery portion of the blood after coagulation. Serum is almost identical to plasma, except that one clotting element is removed.

serum albumin. A derivative of blood plasma that is useful in the treatment of shock and burn victims.

splenectomy. The surgical removal of the spleen, sometimes required after trauma to the abdomen.

S.T.D. Sexually transmitted disease, such as syphilis, gonorrhea, or AIDS.

stroke. An impairment that occurs, when a portion of the brain loses its continuous supply of blood.

surrogate test. In the absence of a direct test for a specific disease, such as a test for the presence of a virus, an indirect test identifying markers usually associated with that disease must sometimes be used. For example, the current ELISA test for AIDS is a surrogate test, since it detects only antibodies to HIV and not the virus itself. Also called *indirect test*.

syphilis. A disease caused by a spirochete and usually spread through sexual contact, occasionally by blood transfusion.

T-cell (also called *T-lymphocyte*). A special group of white blood cells involved with immunity. The T-cell count is a measure of the state of the body's immune system based on the number of T-lymphocytes in the blood. Loss of T-cells is associated with loss of immunity.

transfusion. A transfer of fluid—blood or saline—into a vein or artery from an outside source.

transplant. A transfer of tissue or body parts from one individual to another.

undertransfusion. The practice of not adequately replacing a patient's blood loss because of fear of contamination.

unit. The basic measurement for various substances used in transfusion. It is not an absolute quantity. For example, a unit of whole blood is a little less than a pint. But a unit of red cells is the amount of red cells in one unit of whole blood. Thus a unit of whole blood contains one unit of red cells, one unit of platelets, and one unit of plasma.

vein. A vessel carrying dark red or unaerated blood to the heart, except for the pulmonary vein, which carries oxygenated blood.

ventricle. One of two pumping chambers in the heart which receive blood from the atrium. The right ventricle pumps blood to the lungs and the left ventricle to all other parts of the body.

volunteers. When used in conjunction with blood donors, people who do not receive payment for donating blood.

white blood cells (also known as *leukocytes*). Cells that are instrumental in fighting bacteria and other diseases by producing antibodies.

window period. A term used to describe the gap between the time when an infection first occurs and when the initial, detectable signs of infection first appear.

Index

211